The Great Weight Debate

Get the Facts and Choose the Diet That's Right For You

Amy Newman Shapiro RD, CDN, CPT

Edited by PJ Dempsey
Cover and interior design by Karen Saunders, KarenSaundersAssoc.com
Printed in the United States of America
First Printing: 2021
ISBN: 978-0-9886071-2-5
Library of Congress Control Number: 2020915518

For my grandchildren

In a world where you can be anything, be truthful, trustworthy, courageous, and kind. But most of all, be healthy.

CONTENTS

PART THREE: GETTING HEALTHY/STAYING HEALTHY

Acknowledgments

Throughout the writing of this book, I have been fortunate to have family and friends cheering me on, providing emotional support and technological assistance. Many thanks to Dana Shapiro for her cheerleading, critical eye, wisdom, and infinite patience. Thank you to Carrie Fleishman for your friendship, and for cleaning up my grammatical errors and typos. To Nancy Newman, whose creativity and commitment to detail helps every one of my projects come to life. To Kate Flaxman, thank you for being my inspiration to forge ahead even in the toughest of times. I am forever thankful to my husband, Mitch, for endless encouragement, support, humor, and our happily ever after. I am grateful to my editor, PJ Dempsey, whose enthusiasm and talent turned my manuscript into a book worth reading. I would not have this book in hand without the efforts and creativity of Karen Saunders at Karen Saunders & Associates. Finally, my deepest thanks to all who kept me grounded and cared for during the dark days of the Covid-19 pandemic.

Thank you for reading.

Introduction

Successful weight loss has been a hot topic for years. My first presentation on the subject was in 2004. In fact, it was my first lecture in front of a large audience, ever. At the time, even though it was before the surge in use of social media, the posting of the video of that presentation was viewed all over the country, a testament to the interest in the subject. Subsequent videos of my performances as a lecturer have improved but the universal battle over the bulge has not. Years have passed and people are still searching for a method that will help them lose weight and keep it off. Fifty-eight percent of adults in a survey done by U.S. Center for Disease Control and Prevention answered yes to trying to lose weight in the past year.

More than half the U.S. adult population is trying to lose weight, but few are succeeding. The answer to how to achieve long-term weight loss is not straightforward or simple. As a registered dietitian nutritionist, integrative and functional nutrition practitioner, and certified personal trainer, I have helped people achieve lasting weight loss in private practice, counseling individuals and developing and implementing group weight loss programs. This book is an extension of my knowledge gained over the years. How to lose weight is the topic of numerous conversations, articles, and television programs. It is distressing to know so many people are putting time and effort into a method that will disappoint them or put their health at risk. Weight loss is inextricably tied to health and yet, in this day and age, dieting is a business and the advice is not necessarily coming from health professionals.

Frankly, there are few resources available to help evaluate all the information encountered. I saw a way to help people sift through the minefield of recommendations and misinformation to choose the best diet for success and wrote this incredibly useful manual for anyone considering going on a diet.

Because of the escalation of health issues caused by poor food choices, people are looking at their food intake (that is, food and drink regularly provided or consumed), not only from a weight loss perspective, but also how a diet may help resolve concerns such as uncontrolled blood sugar, high cholesterol, reflux, thyroid disease, and fatigue.

Today, there is a great interest in wellness, not just weight loss... with a focus on how we feel, how to choose foods to increase energy, and how to reduce risk of disease, making it even more essential to choose healthy methods to reach your weight and wellness goals.

To date, some diet trends have supportive research to back up their methodology and claims. There are some popular diets and also other diets that few hear about that are effective and present a healthy way to achieve sustainable weight loss. There are many to choose from with new diets being introduced in the media all the time. Media, including books, blogs, and news reports drives interest in specific diets...after all, weight loss is big business. The diet industry is making billions, $70 billion a year by most recent reports, often with misleading claims and unhealthy practices. Fad diets, fashionable weight loss plans that promise big results but rarely deliver, are all over the media. The loudest voices in the weight debate are often celebrities, influencers, and spokespeople with little or no professional training in weight loss or health, and no scientific research to support their platform.

There are many individual factors that influence how successful you will be with any one method, which is partly the reason people rarely enjoy the results their diet claims to inspire. When choosing a fad diet or weight-loss trend, it is important to select the one that is right for you, keeping your individual health and genomic profile in mind (see Nutrigenomics pg. 123). For the best outcomes, you need to choose a diet that includes your food preferences and meets the needs of your lifestyle, schedule, and food availability. You also need to know how a weight loss plan will impact your health. It is important to put health first, at any weight. By focusing on overall health at any size, success can be measured by more than just a number on the scale. Improvements in energy, digestion, blood pressure, and mood can be celebrated.

The connection between physical health and weight is a big one. A healthier body loses weight more easily. Optimal nutrition rarely exists with a diet that deprives the body of a food group or sufficient calories. Restrictive diets can rob you of energy, weaken bones, and harm vital body functions. But some diets can help you lower blood sugar, lipid levels, or blood pressure. Still others can help you identify food sensitivities. Choosing a diet should include knowledge of the potential health benefits and risks.

The Great Weight Debate summarizes many of the popular weight loss plans, explains the principles for each diet, provides the research available, and highlights factors that will make it a healthy choice. Discover and understand which diet has too many food restrictions, which diets are easy to use when travelling, how much structure a particular diet provides, and in general the rules you will need to follow. You then have all the information to make an informed decision.

Whether you choose Paleo, low carbohydrate, intermittent fasting, Whole30, or Mediterranean, do it with knowledge and realistic expectations. Learn strategies to use to determine which diet is right for you, which diet may be harmful considering your health risks, what to do when weight loss plateaus, and strategies for weight maintenance. Read up on the new trends, the latest buzz, and the results of the most up-to-date research the experts—those with academic degrees and professional organizations sharing their knowledge and opinion— have to offer. Using a diet may not be the best way to lose weight, but if you are going to make the attempt, know that you choose wisely to get the most out of your efforts.

One reason that trying to lose weight is so confusing and frustrating is that everywhere we turn we see headlines, television shows, and new studies touting weight and weight loss plans…and incredible results. Let's face it, all we want is the solution. In today's world, with so many options to lose weight, every one of them claiming miraculous results, it's impossible to know which ones work and which ones can hurt.

This book will spell that out for you. What I intend to do in the following pages is to use published research wherever possible to support or refute a diet's claims. This way you can be guided by facts and experts—not celebrities and product manufacturers—for healthy dieting information.

A Note To The Reader

The diets highlighted within these pages are not all-encompassing but, to the best of my ability, I included the most popular diets and those that tend to raise many questions. There is no significance to the order in which the diets are presented or the extent to which they are reviewed. Rest assured, however, that I included as much information as I could find for each weight-loss method.

The entries vary in length simply because some diets needed more explanation than others. The diets are not ordered by their success rates, or in similarity of methodology, and this was intentional. The material, or the way it is presented, is not meant to steer you in a particular direction, only to make it easy for you to choose your own path. Mentioning one diet first doesn't mean it's the best.

Use the table of contents to locate the page number of a specific diet or food trend. You will find an explanation of the diet, scientific research, and expert opinion if available to support the choice, and also a quick reference guide of the key points to consider in the decision to give it a try or pass it by. To round out your research on this important topic, don't miss the chapters on what nutrition experts and scientists recommend for smart eating, and strategies for successful weight loss and keeping it off.

There is no one correct way to lose weight and, in fact, it may take several weight loss methods to reach a goal weight. *The Great Weight Debate* can be used to examine the variety of possible weight loss methods or to use the manual as a reference to become familiar with one particular diet. My hope is that in providing easy to use summaries of the most popular diets and current trends, I provide you the essential material to making an informed decision ultimately leading to long-lasting weight loss.

PART ONE:
WEIGHT LOSS 101

Chapter 1:
The Big Business
Of Marketing And Selling Diets

The diet industry is a seventy-billion-dollar enterprise that keeps growing each year and it is easy to see why. As the money pours in from weight loss foods and supplements, dieting programs, and the next best diet books, the diet industry is expanding its net worth as fast as the rest of us are expanding our waistlines. According to the World Health Organization's last complete year of worldwide statistics, 1.9 billion adults were overweight in 2016, with 650 million classified as obese. This frightening number also translated into sixty percent of the population of the U.S. needing to lose weight, with over 37% classified as obese. As you've probably guessed, these statistics have only gotten worse in the years since.[1]

Public health institutions have not provided clear and adequate weight loss solutions, allowing businesses with no health experts or scientific testing to fill the void. Marketing strategies that play on our feelings of guilt and shame, and insecurities about body image push us to sign up for weight loss and fitness programs, and to spend money to follow the latest diet in the hope of relieving those bad feelings. Evidence of this phenomenon is witnessed in the surge in advertising and media attention to weight loss in January after holiday overindulging and in the Spring, threatening the arrival of swimsuit season, a wedding or high school reunion.

The bookstore shelves, lined with diet books from those who have the best credentials and those who just think they do, add to the abundance of weight loss suggestions on the internet and through social media. What you have is a combination of influencers, with no authenticity, able to reach an unsuspecting public who have no real way to evaluate what they are being sold. Since weight is a health issue, as is high blood pressure and diabetes that often follows, weight loss should not be a profit-centered business, without public welfare as the mission, but should be in the hands of health care professionals. At the very least, diet strategies should be vetted, and either approved or rejected by science, much like food label claims, before being allowed to circulate among media outlets.

Compounding the scarcity of reliable sources of information concerning effective weight loss is the fact that, to date, most physicians have no education in nutrition. Most patients report there is no conversation about weight during yearly physicals, and in the cases where overweight was mentioned, no advice was forthcoming, and no referral was made to a registered dietitian nutritionist.

Many people are not even aware of being overweight. A Gallup poll survey of overweight individuals considered themselves to be at a healthy weight despite the scales proving them otherwise. This, too, may be a byproduct of the population getting heavier because the concept of what being overweight looks like has changed. The number of obese people has increased—it just seems normal to be carrying excess weight—and that is dangerous when it comes to trying to stay healthy. For example, the Diet and Health Knowledge Survey of 1994-1996 found that people who reported their calorie intake as appropriate, were actually overweight or obese, both defined as having an excessive fat accumulation that impairs health.

It's true that valid help can be found on social media where people share experiences and resources. Designed to bring a community of like-minded individuals together, these sites are not always a safe and reliable place for health advice. Keep in mind that weight loss and fitness techniques, which directly impact health, and are being marketed on the internet, are not always appropriate, especially to those who are inexperienced with dieting and exercise.

The weight loss measures marketed by fad diet websites and influencers are often too extreme for the average person to tolerate. Sixty percent of the population is entrenched in unhealthy food practices. It is best not to attempt an all-out diet overhaul that may be daunting and hard to stick with or may have health consequences, and yet, those are the diets with the greatest media exposure and popularity.

The Growth In Popularity Of The Fad Diet

The typical Western Diet that most of us eat in the United States is not considered healthy. It's described as large portions of red meat, processed meats, cheeses, and deep fried foods—all high in fat—along with large helpings of cereals, desserts, breads, salty snack foods, and sweetened drinks that are all high in processed carbohydrates and sugar. What contributes to making this diet even more unhealthy is that it is perilously low in vegetables, fruits, fish, and whole grains. Everything about the Western Diet has contributed to the continued increase in obesity, which has been on the rise for decades.

From 1985 to 2000, there was approximately a 12% increase in the number of calories in the American diet. This is the largest increase ever recorded. Chalk this up to our love of sugary drinks (32 gallons per person in 2011—this is the equivalent of drinking 341 12-oz. cans of soda), dessert consumption (the equivalent of eating 22 teaspoons of sugar per day), and fat-laden cheese consumption (33 pounds per year per person). And Europeans are catching up. The main culprits are convenience and fast foods and their increased levels of fat, sugar, and salt, not to mention huge portion sizes. In 1980, the average drink was 6 ounces and today it is 20 ounces (think super-size and big gulp). Even the average size bagel has grown from 2 ounces to 5-7 ounces.

Kevin Hall, an investigator with the National Institute of Diabetes and Digestive and Kidney Diseases, tells us that since 1980, portion sizes account for an additional 500-800 calories added per day to the average diet. He points out that only eating 50% of these extra calories can account for the rise in obesity.

An increase of 3500 calories can account for a one-pound gain every nine days. If you consider that gaining one pound every nine days translates into 40 pounds more weight in a year, it is easy to see how an increase of 300 calories a day adds up. Eating take-out or fast food at least once or twice a week or eating snack foods with no portion control, and relying on processed foods, are the main sources of these additional calories. A study of over 5,000 employees across the U.S. showed that snacking from vending machines, common areas, meetings, and worksite social events contributed almost 1,300 calories a week in fat, sugar, and refined grains mostly from baked goods, soft drinks, and sandwiches. In addition, the recent shift to work more hours from home puts us in close proximity to our kitchens and more opportunities to snack. Ironically, it seems that eating at work has become an occupational hazard and that many of us are not aware of the extra calories we unconsciously consume during the workday.

We have all heard about the studies linking the Western diet to obesity and the health consequences that go with it. Think about what's going on internally. Obesity leads to heart disease, diabetes, autoimmune and gastrointestinal diseases, hypertension, hyperinsulinemia, osteoarthritis, nonalcoholic fatty liver disease and increased risk of some forms of cancer, not to mention everyday aches and pains (think aching back and knees). With each of these health issues comes the real threat of decreased quality of life and a shorter life span. When you consider that eighty percent of obese adults have *at least one* of these conditions, it's easy to understand how losing weight can save lives.

When obesity was first noted as an epidemic, fad diets became the popular solution. These fad diets were the ones that promised quick weight loss by encouraging dieters to eat what were often unhealthy and imbalanced meals. Fad dieting rules often restricted the foods that contained vital nutrients. Weight loss often consisted of water weight (not fat) leading to a quick regain of weight once the dieting stopped. In addition, the rules and restrictions were not sustainable long-term because they lead to boredom and cravings. The "quick fix" they offered had nothing to do with educating the user in the ways of healthy eating, so old habits and poor food choices returned as did the weight. Fad diets, with extreme restrictions, are still around today and their health risks far outweigh any of the health benefits from the weight loss they produce. To make matters worse, there are even long-term problems resulting from nutrient deficiencies including osteoporosis, kidney stones, gout, in addition to short-term issues that include constipation, headaches, and impaired athletic performance. Many fad diets have not been around long enough to be scientifically studied or to produce any evidence to support them. Some also market special foods or supplements they require you to purchase.

7

I am assuming you are reading this book because you are contemplating losing weight. It doesn't matter if you are dieting for the first time or are a veteran of many diet approaches. If your goal is to lose weight you need to find the dieting program that not only works, *but it works for you.* A good place to start is with an understanding of how all the excess pounds were gained.

Chapter 2:
Battling The Bulge

To illustrate how detrimental the typical American Diet had become, we watched as obesity spread into countries and cultures, where it was almost non-existent, once typical American foods became available. Immigrants from countries where weight and associated diseases were rare became overweight and obese once they were living in the United States. Our typical American diet is not only high in processed carbohydrates, sugars, unhealthy fats and served in large portions, it also contains fewer vegetables, fruits, and whole grains than meals of other cultures. Basically, Americans overeat everything *except* vegetables and fruits.

We Eat Too Much:
The Post-industrial Post World War II Phenomenon

Consider that the typical dinner plate in 1950 was 9-inches in diameter and that today's plates are 10-12 inches in diameter. Not only are they capable of holding a lot more food, but we tend to load them up to the point where we are used to eating larger portion sizes. Because we consume larger than appropriate portions of food, even healthy food, more than our body needs, it stores this unused energy source as body fat.

For a detailed look at how portion sizes have changed, there are websites available to illustrate.[2]

Nutrition facts on food labels was a big step forward in educating consumers about the fat, added sugar, and calories in what they were about to eat. However, serving sizes listed were up to the discretion of the manufacturer, who used market research to determine how much the average person consumed of that particular product. As people became accustomed to eating more, the serving sizes listed on the package became larger, leading the consumer to eat the larger serving size listed and not by personal hunger level or desire. Larger portions are so expected that now manufacturers will also list the nutrition facts if *you were to eat the entire container.*

Consider, too, how often we eat out today. Growing up in the 1960's, I didn't know what McDonald's was. Now, there's one a block from my office along with a Burger King, Pizza Hut, Panera Bread, Dunkin Donuts, Subway, Chinese take-out, and Starbucks. The average American eats one in every four meals outside the home. Twelve percent of all calories consumed come from fast-food meals. In an effort to win customers with value and quantity, restaurants of every type compete by increasing portion sizes, offering calorie-laden soft drinks loaded with cheap-to-produce forms of sugar.[3]

Another factor leading to weight gain is the decline in physical activity. Modern technology has removed much of our need to move around to get things done. The exercise we used to get from the activities of daily life by performing the household chores of cleaning and laundry, preparing food, walking or bicycling to visit friends or to the store, all burned calories. (Every time I am in an airport, I wonder if it is just a matter of time before moving sidewalks also become commonplace in malls all over America). Because we did not have computers and we spent less time in front of the television, we had time to be more active. Today, too many people think of exercise as a chore. But think about it, instead of sitting and watching YouTube videos and movies, it would be easy to exercise while watching (I have a TV in the basement in front of my treadmill). Sitting is the new smoking in that, like smoking, inactivity contributes to the increased risk of many life-threatening diseases, especially heart disease and diabetes.

Large portions and inactivity are only part of the problem. To find an effective weight loss solution, first you need to learn a few basics about how the body and brain work together in this complicated business of eating, gaining, and losing weight.

Weight-Loss Basics: Why It's So Tough To Get To And Sustain A Desirable Weight

Biology at Work

The first thing you need to know is that weight is controlled by biological systems of hormones, genes, and brain chemicals that regulate appetite and fat storage. These systems literally signal the brain as to what, when, and how much to eat to maintain the current body weight. This same system is rigged to prevent weight loss. It is an efficient system that has kept us alive since the dawn of humankind. It is still, in many ways, a primitive system driven by signals from fat tissues, the liver, brain, and gastrointestinal tract and is designed solely to keep the body alive in case of famine (starving to death). This is why I say the system is rigged, because in order to lose weight this system needs to be tricked into doing something for which it was not designed. This very efficient system is adept at storing any unused calories as fat and humans are very adept at eating more calories than they burn. Without threat of a famine, it's easy to get and stay overweight in today's world. Tricking the body into losing excess weight is easier said than done because when we do cut back on food, our brains are programmed to decrease metabolism to preserve calories, efficiently putting the brakes on losing body fat.

Blame this dilemma on biology. There are real physical and psychological factors that challenge losing weight in an attempt at self-preservation. The human body has a built-in fail safe against starvation. The body fights to preserve weight much as it does to maintain body temperature. Quick weight loss triggers the brain to fight to replace fat stores and restore lost body weight. Unfortunately, the brain cannot differentiate between intentional weight loss and starvation. Any weight loss also triggers an increase in the production of appetite hormones to restore lost weight, so, just when you start to eat less, hunger levels rise. Successful dieters learn to modify what they eat and how much they eat to outsmart biology.

Diets also cause internal hunger and satiety cues to atrophy because they reprogram us to rely instead on external cues. Weight loss is affected as much by not eating enough as it is by eating too much. This happens because severe calorie restriction slows metabolism, so calories burned slows, and the excess ones are stored as fat. To counter this, experts tell us that eating 1,200 calories a day is the minimum needed to meet energy and reduce the risk of slowed metabolism.

Dieting Leads To Thoughts Of Food

Unfortunately, trying to control all aspects of eating causes the starving and deprived brain to be preoccupied with thoughts of food. This is another biological function designed to counter the effects of famine by constantly reminding us to go find food and to not stop until we do. This is also why dieting even triggers food obsessions, often with foods we don't even usually crave. You are not imagining this—it is how we're built.

Furthermore, we eat what we like, what's available, what is convenient, and when we have the time to eat. We also don't like being told what and what not to eat. Diets remove the ability to eat intuitively. That is why following a diet can lead to feelings of deprivation, cravings, binging, and guilt. The physical and mental dieting challenges act together to lead to feelings of failure when eating forbidden foods. For example, if you aren't in the mood for the diet-prescribed food or it is not available, it is not uncommon to experience stress, anxiety, guilt, and frustration. These negative thoughts and emotions may then lead you to overeat or make more poor choices. Have you ever come home from a party where you didn't eat the food only to sit down with a pint of ice cream? How many times have you thought that since you wrecked your diet anyway that you may as well eat as much as you can and start again on Monday? This diet mentality of using "good" and "bad" labels for foods increases the struggle between following prescribed rules and actual food desires.

Calories Count, Food Quality Too

Excess weight comes from eating calorie-dense foods too frequently or portion sizes that are too big. Controlling portions can actually permit you to eat even the high-calorie foods typically forbidden on weight-loss diets, and still lose weight or maintain weight.[4] Keep in mind that the serving size listed in nutrition facts on food labels is based on how much people eat and not how much they **should** eat. This means that manufacturers adjust the serving size based on current trends in eating habits. As our portion sizes have increased over the years, food companies have also increased the serving sizes. These changes can mislead you to eat more of a food than is wise. But what you choose to eat is yet another important factor when managing weight.

The currency of weight is calories, yet weight loss success also depends on how these calories are spent. In a *New York Times* opinion piece September 2012, Dr. Dean Ornish, professor of medicine at the University of California and founder of Preventative Medicine Research Institute, wrote "Perhaps the biggest misconception is that as long as you lose weight, it doesn't matter what you eat. But it does." It would be impossible to lose weight and sustain the weight loss if you consistently ate meals of burgers with fries and bagels with cream cheese, topped off with cookie snacks, even if you did stay within a calorie allotment. Processed carbohydrates and high-fat proteins (beef and cheese for example), without vegetables and fruits have been shown to be ineffective. By focusing on whole foods (full of filling fiber and water) and getting rid of processed foods (full of fat and sugar), you can cut 500 calories out of your day. Consider planning your daily allotment of calories as you do to plan your financial budget. You use money for rent and utilities before spending money on clothes and movies. So too, spend your daily calories on fruits, vegetables, whole grains, and healthy fats before you splurge on fast food, ice cream, and sugary drinks.

The Impact Of Sleep And Stress

You need mental energy and focus when you are trying to lose or maintain weight. Stress and lack of sleep both sap energy and impact brain and body function. Stress also causes many people metabolic hormonal changes that result in inflammation and increased cortisol, the hormone that affects blood sugar and fat storage. Stress also messes with the hormones that control hunger and satiety.

Sleep quality also affects our weight. Snoring and sleep apnea, which interrupts sleep, increases risk of obesity, unless treated. Blue light emitted from televisions, lamps, and personal devices used in bed interfere with quality of sleep and raises the likelihood of gaining weight. Many electronic devices are equipped with a setting to block this type of sleep-disturbing light. If yours has one, take advantage of it and use it. Sleep patterns influence eating habits and eating habits influence sleep. Sleep-impaired people eat more and make poor food choices. And there is evidence that backs this up. When we don't get enough sleep, fat intake increases. Other evidence links high-fat diets to insomnia, proving that food habits affect sleep and sleep affects food habits. Also, when scientists looked at protein intake, they found that people sleeping less than seven hours ate less protein and more carbohydrates. This is not surprising, since the brain, short on sleep and therefore energy, wants more of its preferred form of fuel. Additionally, a protein-rich meal is more satisfying, therefore, consuming less of it often leads to eating larger portions of carbohydrates and fat. More evidence of how food affects sleep was found in a Japanese study where a low protein diet, less than 19% of total calories, was linked to trouble falling asleep as well as poor sleep quality. Research on the relationship between carbohydrates and sleep quality, though, is less clear. It appears that eating both too little and too much in the way of carbs is associated with poor sleep quality. Eating more fiber is associated with better sleep while eating high sugar foods and highly processed carbs is linked to poor sleep. This translates to eating processed carbohydrates like bread, pasta and sugary snacks affecting sleep negatively compared to whole grains and produce. Both caffeine and alcohol impact sleep. It is not just how much is consumed but what time of day. Any way you look at it, carefully choosing what you eat and drink has a major influence on sleep and weight.

The Mind At Work

There is the mindset that including attitude and the mental energy it takes to find new ways to eat keeps thoughts positive, make healthy food decisions and choose healthy behaviors.

The key to making healthy food decisions and lifestyle choices is mindfulness. Mindful eating is a nonjudgmental awareness of the nurturing aspects of food selection and preparation; choosing foods without censorship that are satisfying, enjoyable, and nutritious; paying attention to the physical sensations of eating including all the senses; and being guided by internal cues of hunger and fullness, which signal the body when to eat and when to stop.

Mindful eating:
- ✓ Reduces calorie intake
- ✓ Increases weight loss
- ✓ Reduces out-of-control eating
- ✓ Increases enjoyment of food
- ✓ Promotes control of food choices and portion sizes
- ✓ Encourages awareness of thoughts and feelings about food

Being mindful and intentional about what, when, and how you eat includes preplanning healthy meals, eating slowly to allow the body to signal when it's full, and removing the television, computer, and all other non-eating distractions from mealtime. Paying attention without distractions when eating meals and snacks leads to feeling satisfied with less. What is gained by adopting this behavior is less time and mental energy wasted on eating. Meal planning, grocery shopping, and putting a meal together should be the only time spent focusing on food.

Unfortunately, dieting stirs up many emotions. We rely on virtuosity, willpower, and good/bad comparisons, and when the diet doesn't go as planned, we feel shame and guilt. Fad diets are marketed to appeal to our insecurities concerning body image and lifestyle. Shame and guilt get in the way of feeling happy and healthy. Dieting can also lead to decreased self-esteem as well as anxiety and even depression. Dieters often become a slave to the scale, determining their self-worth by a number. These thoughts and emotions negatively impact the energy and effort needed to make healthy decisions and lifestyle changes, adding to the struggle to lose weight.

Successful weight loss often depends on identifying and addressing emotional eating. Stress eating, binge eating, and eating from boredom or loneliness are ways we use food to soothe our emotions. Eating, without hunger, for comfort is a habit contributing to overweight/obesity. Often therapy is helpful to end this unhealthy relationship with food.

I hope you can see now how nutrition affects mood, emotional state, energy level, and health. Losing weight is easier when you are happy, positive, full of energy, and emotionally healthy.

Yes, you can lose weight and keep it off by dieting. Think of it as the best way to impose structure to your eating by way of a plan. Choose a diet that teaches you how to successfully manipulate foods you enjoy, employing healthy behaviors, in such a way that leads to weight loss. This is how to have the best chance at enjoying permanent weight loss.

Healthy Dieting for Permanent Weight Loss

Permanent weight loss can only happen when lasting lifestyle changes are made. Even small changes in food intake or physical activity contribute toward permanent weight loss. Performing small changes that are doable and sustainable work because they generate feelings of accomplishment that are both motivating and capable of encouraging even more changes. Short-term efforts, like concentrating on moderating portion sizes and making healthier food choices, have a cumulative effect that over time creates the lifestyle changes that result in permanent weight loss. Making small incremental adjustments consistently over time means no struggle. It is how new healthy habits are established.

Habits

A habit is a behavior we perform without thought. The word *habit* has a negative connotation for many people because we associate it with undesirable behaviors including overeating. But you now need to think of habits as a way to change for the better, replacing those that have gotten you to this place with their counterparts that will get you to your new healthy place. We need habits, but we need good ones.

Establishing a new habit takes thought, planning, and fortitude—and it's easier than you think. Repeatedly performing a new behavior, instead of the old one, is what creates a new habit.

The good news is that it only takes 3 weeks to 3 months to form a new habit when you have a supportive environment, both physical and social. Even the best efforts can be sabotaged by well-meaning friends, spouses, or work environments offering tempting foods. But, if you are aware of these pitfalls, you can sidestep them, at least until your new habits are firmly established. And once that new habit becomes part of your everyday experience, you can feel proud because it means a lifestyle change has occurred.

Realistic Goals Are Achievable Goals

Any new habit that changes the way you eat and burn calories is a small positive step in your everyday life that will lead you to your weight goal and keep you there. With small steps that relate to your weight and health goals, you realize short-term successes that help you achieve permanent change, which in turn leads to achieving lifetime goals. You climb stairs one at a time, achieving a major goal happens the same way. The more realistic and attainable the goal, the more likely you are to put in the effort and accomplish it. If climbing stairs leaves you breathless, training for a marathon is unrealistic, but a daily walk with the dog is a good start. If you have children to get ready for school, planning to get to the gym before 8 AM is not a realistic goal. Likewise, if you really enjoy eating chips, choosing not to eat them anymore is unrealistic, but eating them less often and in much smaller portions is a realistic and achievable goal. Goals also must be specific in terms of both an identifiable task and setting a detailed time frame to complete it. Instead of simply saying your goal is to avoid the vending machine at work, say your task is to take a fruit or yogurt to work with you to eat for a snack at 3:00 PM.

Goals also need to be measurable to be accountable for their completion and also to identify and celebrate each achievement. Food journals, pedometers, portion-controlled bowls and utensils, and exercise logs are all ways to evaluate performance.

Don't Be Ruled (Or Fooled) By The Scale

All too often, dieting success or failure is determined by the number you see on the scale. Don't fall for it. The weight registered on the scale is affected by many, often temporary, factors including fluid retention, salt intake, and hormone shifts. Keep in mind, too, that not every temporary increase in weight is bad. An increase in physical activity increases muscle mass, for example, meaning improved body composition that will increase metabolism and lead to weight loss in the long-term, but the short-term effect often appears to be a weight gain on the scale. So, you see, the scale is not always a true indicator of fat loss at that moment and is certainly not a true measure of health. Having more energy or a lower blood pressure reading are significant achievements that cannot be measured on a scale.

But, the scale also reminds us of the pounds that are no longer being added. If the number on your scale has been increasing over the years, reversing the upward trend is an achievement. Adopting new behaviors that put an end to weight gain is cause for celebration or at least a pat on the back.

The results on the scale do help some people to stay focused on new behaviors and goals, and that's great. However, if you find weighing in negatively affecting your self-regard, even if the ups and downs on the scale are unrelated to your choices, then don't weigh yourself. The scale is not a barometer of self-worth and using the number on the scale to determine how good you should or should not feel isn't wise or helpful. Negative thoughts lead to negative effort, which leads to negative results. When this happens, the scale ceases to be a useful tool.

If weighing yourself works for you, do it at least once a week to assess progress. Scales with body fat analyzers may be of interest, although not highly accurate in assessing improvement in body composition (fat loss).

Reward Yourself

Whatever helps you assess, acknowledge, and reward your positive behavior and lifestyle changes is the one sure way to see results. Choosing non-food treats to look forward to after reaching a short-term goal is a powerful motivator to stick to your diet and exercise goals. Plan a movie, a massage or even time with a book and a cup of tea. The idea is to find a way to pat yourself on the back for a job well done.

Yo-Yo Dieting

Yo-yo dieting is the endless cycle of losing and regaining weight. It is the unhealthy consequence that happens when diets don't work long-term and it is very common. The reason why is that most diets focus on limiting or eliminating specific food groups or targeted foods, along with rules governing timing of meals and snacks. But this approach is difficult to sustain. Accompanying the lower number on the scale are feelings of accomplishment and pride. With those feelings, deprivation is challenging to sustain, effort to follow rules wanes. But this is only a temporary win because when people stop abiding by the rules and restrictions, returning to old eating habits, lo and behold, the pounds that took so much effort to lose not only return, but often bring with them even more. Once again, the dieting begins, weight is lost and regained, and the yo-yo weight cycle continues. The only thing that breaks this cycle is a weight loss method that creates permanent change in food behaviors and lifestyle to sustain both weight loss and weight maintenance.

Long-Term Weight Loss Takes Time

Be realistic, it may have taken months or years to put the weight on and expecting to lose it in a short amount of time is setting yourself up for failure. When we don't meet our goal, we tend to feel negative about ourselves, including our efforts or the methods we chose. So always be realistic about your initial weight goal and remember that the healthiest weight loss is gradual: one to two pounds per week. For someone who is overweight or obese, a total weight loss of ten percent is a realistic goal. Once this goal is achieved you can always set a second goal. Remember, this is not a race. As long as the weight is coming off (even a half pound is significant) it means the behaviors you have chosen are working for you. Being realistic about how much you can lose also decreases disappointment. Disappointment leads to less effort. Less effort leads to fewer results, which perpetuates the negative feelings.

It is also important to sustain the same food and lifestyle changes after reaching your goal as the main strategy for maintaining your weight loss. After all, if a particular weight loss strategy helped you to lose five pounds, repeating the same method will likely result in another five pounds gone. This way you can more easily lose weight in five-pound increments, if you aren't concerned about how long it takes.

There is a lot of controversy and impassioned discussion concerning how people choose to try to lose weight. There is no one size fits all diet, no cookie cutter solution. The answer may be the best diet for you is the one that fits your lifestyle and food preferences so that you will stick with it.[5]

PART TWO:
THE DIETS

Chapter 3:

Popular Diets —
The Good, The Bad,
And The Just Plain Hungry

This book should dispel many of the myths and misinformation you've heard or read concerning the most popular diets. In addition, it is designed to provide you with the knowledge you need to choose the healthiest and best alternative for you. It is my intent that highlighting the good, the bad, and the ugly of each diet will give you a head-start to success with any of the weight loss methods you choose. As much as I've tried my best to make sure that these descriptions are totally inclusive of every aspect of each diet, that is just not possible. However, my research should serve as enough of an overview to help you identify the weight loss method you wish to follow. I have endeavored to include the most current research available up to the time of publication. Do keep in mind that results from efficacy studies of most diets vary widely, which means you will read differing opinions, some supporting and some refuting a particular method or finding. I suggest you use this information as you would when reading any type of review and simply decide which opinion resonates with you. After all, if the diet doesn't end up working for you, you can always switch to another one.

I have evaluated the weight loss plans I feel represent the range of different types that appeal to today's lifestyle. Besides, it would have been impossible to cover every diet due to the number of new ones appearing almost monthly in the media and in books. If you are interested in seeing what is on the horizon, see page 105 for trending strategies and the latest research.

It is especially important that you keep in mind that some diets are more effective for some dieters than others. This is due, in part, to genetics or even to factors related to environment or lifestyle. Also, of utmost importance to dietary success is that the people who are most successful at losing weight and keeping it off have used several programs. This changing of parameters and restrictions every few weeks or months works to decrease boredom and permits the guilt-free eating of favorite foods. We've found that sometimes loosening restrictions works best to support optimal nutrition and, ultimately, better health. So, when choosing one of the many roads on your journey to wellness, make sure you allow yourself to change course if a diet plan is making you miserable or isn't getting results. Choose a new road when weight loss stops or the pounds start piling on again. When you find a healthy weight loss method that is working for you, stick to it for 4-6 months. Then stop it and maintain the weight you reached for another 4-6 months and repeat. Pausing along the way gives your metabolism and behavior a chance to adjust and helps to keep from triggering the unhealthy practice of yo-yo dieting. I have clients who have used unrealistic, unsustainable methods to lose the same weight, up to 100 pounds, more than once.

Losing weight is a difficult task. Acknowledge that fact. Choose a realistic goal and celebrate the small successes to reduce frustration and keep you motivated. Choosing an eating plan you can live with not only makes reaching your weight-loss goal easier, it prevents the cycle of repeatedly losing and regaining the weight.

The High Protein Diet

High protein diet means low in carbohydrates (a.k.a. carbs) and high in protein, and sometimes fat. This type of fad diet gained popularity with the introduction of the Atkins diet more than 30 years ago followed by several others, including The South Beach and Zone diets, which used similar diet restrictions. A current internet search yielded 7,320,000 results for 'high protein diet plan,' so you can see the popularity remains. Although there are no specific guidelines for what a high protein diet actually means, the Institute of Medicine does recommend that adults should consume 0.8 grams of protein per kilogram (kg) of body weight (to convert your body weight from pounds to kilograms, simply divide by 2.2). For an adult weighing 150 lbs., adequate protein would be 55 grams per day, roughly 15% of total daily calorie intake. US Dietary Reference Intakes sets an upper limit for protein consumption at 35% of total calorie intake (for an 1,800-calorie diet that is 157 grams). Although most adults consume more than the 15% minimum protein requirement, protein needs do vary among adults, depending on gender, activity level, and body composition. For example, those who body-build or perform endurance sports and pregnant women need more.

This type of diet imposes a carbohydrate restriction, which means the two macronutrients left to provide adequate calories are fats and protein. Even though fats no longer take the rap for all the health ills befalling us, the whopping calories they do contain—whether as healthy fats or not—should still dissuade you from increasing fats to more than 30% of your total daily calories without guidance from a physician or registered dietitian. Done right, eating more protein is a healthier way of reducing carbohydrate consumption.

How It Works

How high protein diets cause weight loss:
- Protein intake during weight loss preserves lean body mass (muscle) and maintains metabolism.

- Protein keeps you feeling fuller longer because protein-rich foods take longer to digest, increase production of satiety hormones (chemical messengers that make you feel you've had enough), and reduce levels of hunger hormones, lowering total calorie intake.

- High protein foods use more calories to process so the body burns more calories digesting them.

- Weight maintenance is easier after successful high protein dieting, although the jury is still out as to whether this outcome is dependent on individual genetics.

What The Experts Say

Initial reports are promising that higher protein diets do help with weight loss but the scientific research backing these claims isn't there just yet. Studies also attribute additional health benefits including reduction in LDL (bad) cholesterol along with the reduced carbohydrate intake, as well as a 30% reduction in the risk of heart disease. But these results may be more dependent on choosing lean protein food sources, including fish, turkey, and chicken, as well as vegetable protein (legumes, beans, nuts, and soy), and reducing intake of beef and processed meats.

Fad diets with the emphasis on high protein do not usually result in sustainable long-term weight loss. The restrictions these diets place on eating and lifestyle are hard to maintain and, since portion size and calorie intake are not addressed during weight loss, the pounds return when the restrictions are lifted.

Reasons to Avoid High Protein Diets:

- Temporary weight loss, often with more weight regained than lost

- Initial weight loss is from water, not body fat

- Consumption of more animal protein, including processed/deli meats means more saturated fat, chemicals, and microbes

- This diet tends to be deficient in the fiber, antioxidants, vitamins/minerals that are important to sustain health

- Evidence that a high protein diet puts added stress on kidney function in certain individuals

Remember that eating too much protein, like eating too many carbs or too much fat, also contributes to excess calories being turned into body fat. Keep an eye on your caloric bottom line. If high protein means high in calories, this will not help you lose weight. Also, don't believe the false claims that a high protein diet helps you build muscle. Weight training is what builds muscle strength. Eating protein does aid in muscle recovery, but that may be more to do with **when** you eat the protein rather than the amount you eat.

Is This Diet For You?

Worth A Try: High protein diets can be a good option if you are challenged by high carbohydrate consumption. Eating this way is a good technique to help you rethink your plate and intake of processed grains and starchy vegetables. A high protein diet is fine to follow short-term but consider the foods you will be doing without before you choose it long-term. This diet is a good alternative if switching to another type of diet is part of your plan for continued weight loss or weight maintenance.

Pass It By: High protein diets are not for anyone with impaired liver or kidney function or kidney disease. Before considering this diet, consult your health care provider.

A Closer Look: The Atkins Diet, Wheat Belly, Grain Brain, and The Make-It-Up-As-You-Go Low-Carb Diet

There are so many conflicting ideas as to what constitutes a low carb diet. A good-health rule of thumb is that 40-50% of your total daily calories should be from carbohydrates. However, there is another school of thought that says low carb eating means consuming less than 100 grams of carbs a day. As you will see, common to the diets that follow is the reduction in carbohydrates, however, the severity of the restriction may differ. No matter which one you choose, a physician or registered dietitian needs to be consulted in order to guide you to your healthiest carbohydrate restriction, based on your individual health profile. This is because the degree to which a person can restrict carbohydrate intake for weight loss varies among dieters. Also, from a purely social perspective, a severe carbohydrate restriction has a greater impact on your lifestyle and social calendar and, have no doubt about it, will be less tolerated by friends and family who won't be happy about taking more time and effort to feed you—which plays a major role in why extreme dieting often fails.

Over the years I've met with many people who follow their own ideas of what constitutes a low carbohydrate diet. It's amazing that nearly all these low-carb dieters are either unaware or uninformed as to how many sources of carbohydrates exist in various foods. In my professional experience, the most misguided and extreme attempt at low-carb dieting was a client who claimed to be eating a carb-free diet for the past year, per her doctor's orders. She had indeed removed all carbohydrate containing foods from her meals, however, she snacked on brownies two times a day! Needless to say, her weight loss method was not successful.

It is so much more than just eliminating bread, pasta, and the like from your plate. Your choice of which carbs you continue to eat is important too. For example, dieters who consumed a variety of healthy fruits, vegetables, and whole grains in moderate portions and avoided processed and packaged starches enjoyed successful weight loss and healthy outcomes. Conversely, those who favored a more severe carbohydrate restriction were prone to binges or frequent weekend over-consuming. This attempt at a non-sustainable change in food choices or portion sizes also translated to a non-sustainable weight loss.

The body needs carbohydrates and carbohydrates are pervasive in our food supply, so it is important to point out just how many foods fall into this important nutrient category. To be clear, foods like fruits, vegetables, milk, and yogurt contain carbohydrates without impact on our weight, especially since the water content in these carbs means you can eat them in a larger volume while ingesting fewer calories—which translates into feeling fuller with less food. So, more food, more nutrients, less calories, less hunger, why would you want to eliminate these carbs??

I don't believe carbohydrates should be labeled good or bad. The truth is that even "good" carbs are "bad" if consumed in large quantities. That is why portion control is really the important key to weight loss and weight maintenance. Often, it is more about how much you eat, not what you eat, that determines the size of your waist.

Use Caution Around These Carbs

The following sources of carbohydrates are easy to overeat:

- Bagels/Bread/Rolls/Muffins/Wraps

- Cookies/Cakes/Candy/Ice Cream

- Pasta/Rice/Quinoa/Oats

- Potatoes/Corn/Cassava

- Beans/Lentils/Peas/Soy

- Cereal/Crackers

- Chips/Popcorn

- Soda/Sweetened Iced Tea

- High Fructose Corn Syrup/Table Sugar/Honey/Agave

- Potato Starch/Rice Starch/Corn Starch

Grains are carbohydrates and all you hear these days is to add whole grains to your diet because they are a healthy source of fiber and nutrients. In spite of which low-carb diet philosophy you follow, for your health as well as your weight, replace processed grains with whole grains. Here the message is: the specific foods containing carbs you are eating is as important as how much you eat.

What The Experts Say

Unfortunately, science has not provided clear answers about the efficacy and safety of low-carb dieting. Studies determined that low-carb diets improve blood sugar control in people with diabetes. There are studies showing low-carb dieting has a healthy effect on lipid levels, while others find it negatively impacts LDL "bad" cholesterol and heart function. In spite of the controversy, dieters continue to be attracted to them.

When following a low carbohydrate diet, there needs to be an increase in either protein or fat for adequate energy and to satisfy hunger. A growing body of research indicates 30 grams of protein per meal is enough to improve appetite control, satiety, and weight management. That averages to 20% of total calories, with carbohydrates and fat making up the rest of the total daily calories. Eating adequate protein is also important while dieting to preserve lean body mass (muscle) that the body can break down and use for fuel in the absence of enough protein and calories from food. Consuming protein at every meal helps direct breakdown of body fat instead of muscle. Raising fat intake, however, is another story. Most long-term studies show that fat intake of 30% of total calories promotes a healthy weight and healthy body. Diets that encourage higher fat intake can negatively affect the health of the liver and gallbladder. The best approach is moderation. Lower carbohydrate, not low-carbohydrate intake, limited fat intake, and an adequate amount of lean protein is the best approach.

The newest research from the Framingham State Food Study found eating a lower carbohydrate diet following weight loss helps keep weight off. Weight loss causes major changes in the body, particularly a slower metabolism. By following a plan with total calories appropriate to maintain weight, but choosing 30-40% of calories from carbs, instead of the typical 60-65%, you potentially increase metabolic rate and burn 100-200 more calories. The lower the carbs the more calories burned. Keep in mind the body is healthiest without severe restrictions so aim for a moderate carbohydrate restriction of 30-40% of total daily calories. On an 1800 calorie diet, carbohydrate intake at 30% is 135 grams; on 1300 calories 40% carbs is 130 grams, sufficient for a healthy body and mind.[6]

Is This Diet For You?

Low carbohydrate diets usually show remarkable results in the beginning, depending on the severity of the carbohydrate restriction. Without carbohydrates from food, the body first uses up its stored carbohydrates, also known as glycogen. Glycogen stores include water, a lot of water. Initial weight loss on low carb diets is not only from body fat, but water stores—3-4 pounds of it, which will return as soon as carbs are reintroduced. Celebrating any weight loss success with a carb splurge is counterproductive and can set any weight loss back to the beginning weight almost immediately. Therefore, it is critical to long-term success to wisely choose a plan you can stick with. *Extremely* low carbohydrate diets are a quick fix, not a long-term solution.

Worth a Try: Though it might be temporary, you may lose weight. At a sustainable low-carb level, it may be a good option for weight maintenance too. For optimal health, keep the vegetables, fruits, and whole grains in your diet and avoid overly processed carbs often found in meals and snacks.

Pass It By: If your big picture includes more than a quick small adjustment in your weight, pass it by. Consult a doctor first if you have health issues involving the heart or blood sugar, are pregnant, or at an advanced age.

Atkins Diet

In 1972, Dr. Robert Atkins dramatically altered the dieter's plate with the publication of his book *Dr. Atkins' Diet Revolution.*[7] The Atkins Diet prescribed a drastic reduction in consumption of all sources of carbohydrates in favor of unlimited consumption of protein and fats. During the Atkins heyday it became commonplace to see people eating the burger and tossing the bun. Bacon and butter were consumed in large quantities and often while plant-based foods were totally off the menu. Large helpings of bacon, steak, cheese, greens, and a few other low-carbohydrate vegetables made up this limited diet. At the outset, Atkins followers lost weight quickly, but from water loss, and not from loss of body fat.

How It Works

Atkins recommended carbohydrate intake for the first two weeks at 20 grams of "net carbs" daily, followed by a carbohydrate consumption of no more than 40 grams per day. "Net carbs" was a phrase coined by food companies to make foods appear to be lower in carbohydrates. It is calculated by subtracting the total number of grams of fiber in the food from the total number of carbohydrates in that food. While it is true our bodies don't digest the fiber, the natural bacteria residing in our gut does, and we absorb those calories, making the term "net carbs" misleading. The diet allowed eating unlimited protein and fat and promised quick weight loss, up to 15 lbs. in the first two weeks, although Dr. Atkins did admit that results varied.

Carbohydrates are what fuels the body and, without this primary source of fuel, the body must rely on fats, both from food and body fat. As a result of this fat metabolism, the liver produces chemical compounds called ketones, and the condition caused by producing them is ketosis. Ketones are an alternative energy source created by the breakdown of fat for fuel and their presence tends to reduce appetite, quite a perk when food intake is restricted. (You will find more information on ketosis under Ketogenic diet on page 47).

Ketosis is a biological back-up system and is not suggested as a long-term energy source because ketones increase the body's acidity, which is a pro-inflammatory state with medical implications including brain fog, diarrhea, back pain, insomnia, and rashes. Those who follow Atkins also complain of low energy and rightly so because they are low on carbohydrates, the fuel of the body and for the brain. This is also why those following an extremely low carbohydrate diet often suffer from headaches (60%), constipation (68%), bad breath (38%), and muscle cramps (35%). The nutrient deficiencies in this type of diet also increase the risk of developing osteoporosis and kidney stones.

The human body needs a minimum of 130 grams of carbohydrates each day for its systems to perform optimally. A healthy change in the Atkins Diet is that it now offers two diet plans, the original with a phase 1 restriction to 20 grams of carbohydrates a day, and a second plan that starts the user at 40 g carbs per day. A more liberal approach, this Atkins 40 plan includes carbohydrates from all food groups and is less likely to trigger severe adverse reactions. Also, Atkins now encourages eating more high fiber vegetables. Another update appeared in early 2016 with a shift in focus from big and quick results to realistic and sustainable goals. These changes make the current Atkins platform healthier than the original, but you need to remain wary of their marketing claims. Atkins Nutritionals continues to promote a product line they claim is geared toward the trend of less-processed foods. However, as of this writing, contrary to those claims, these products remain highly processed alternatives to whole foods.

A fun fact concerning the low-carb approach to dieting comes by way of some researchers speculating that Atkins was a success because it was boring. The theory is that because dieters derived less pleasure from eating, they no longer ate large quantities. The more variety in our diet, the more food we tend to eat. It turns out that a monotonous diet is good for losing weight, but to counteract the boredom of low-carb dieting, food manufacturers flooded the market with "low-carb" foods from everything from ice cream to snack bars. Restaurants even jumped on this bandwagon with low-carb menu items. Food companies replaced sugar with sugar alcohols, and grains with indigestible fibers, using the term net-carbs to make the food more attractive to the carb-reluctant consumer. There is no agreement on the terms "low-carb" and "net-carb" but these boredom-reducing foods were very attractive to the Atkins dieters and again had them eating these new versions of pastas, breads, chips, and cookies once taboo. These processed "low carb" food alternatives, however, rendered the Atkins Diet less effective in weight loss. Mintel International

Group, a product-tracking company, found these products had just as many calories as the products they were developed to replace. Also common was the notion that these products, mostly snack foods, were okay to consume in larger quantities or more often. Atkins worked, for the most part, because of the elimination of snack and comfort food. These newly created engineered foods shifted the Atkins diet away from its low carbohydrate roots to a diet plan that was only effective if the dieter consumed fewer calories, much like the premise of every other diet. In the short term, Atkins leads to weight loss success mostly because of water loss when carbs are removed, a 3- to 5-pound weight loss is typical the first week, making the dieter feel successful and virtuous. Then things get a bit rocky.

Because the calories consumed on low carbohydrate diets are by way of high protein and/or high-fat intake, and the Atkins Diet does not differentiate between good fats and bad fats, Atkins' followers unknowingly increase risk of developing heart disease. The message here proves that education from a nutrition professional increases the safety factor of any diet. Choosing lean proteins in white meat, poultry, fish, legumes, and healthy fats from nuts, seeds, and avocado may actually promote heart health while losing weight. Keep in mind, too, with no consideration of portion sizes, you may not be eliminating enough calories to lower on the scale.

Once you reach goal weight the Atkin's Diet claims it can help you identify your personal carbohydrate tolerance. However, without learning about appropriate portion sizes of popular carbohydrates like pasta, bread, cereal, and snack foods, again eating carbohydrates will cause weight gain. Atkins is not a diet for permanent weight loss.

What The Experts Say

Research shows more rapid weight loss in the first three months on Atkins' as compared to standard low-calorie diets, but no difference in total weight loss after one year.

Studies support using high-protein low-carbohydrate diets as a short-term way to jump-start weight loss, but not as a long-term eating plan. The medical community continues to research the effects the Atkins Diet has on cholesterol and triglyceride levels. Low carbohydrate diets have been shown to lower triglycerides, but after two years the results are the same as low-fat diets. Proponents of low-carbohydrate diets cite studies showing beneficial effects on obesity and on insulin resistance, a condition that leads to elevated blood sugars and often to Type 2 Diabetes. Again, research shows low-carb diets are no more effective than conventional diets for both obesity and insulin resistance.

Atkins Diet supporters, often becoming fanatics, have glorified the heart healthy results of eating large amounts of bacon and lard while improving their cholesterol profile. Unfortunately, the only study published exclusively on the Atkins diet showed that LDL (bad) cholesterol went up and HDL (good) cholesterol did not rise as expected with weight loss. Free fatty acid levels, which can cause heart arrhythmias, could double.[8]

In a study of Atkins, Weight Watchers, Ornish and Zone (another low carb weight loss plan), changes in LDL and HDL cholesterol were associated with the weight loss not the food on the plan. Interestingly, the greatest weight loss was in those participants following the Ornish Diet, which is low fat, not low carb.[9]

Is This Diet For You?

This is not to say that a **lower**, not a "**low**"-carbohydrate diet is not advantageous. For one thing, most Americans and other cultures consume way more carbohydrates than the minimum healthy recommendation of 130 grams/day. A typical American diet of 1,800 calories a day includes more than 250 grams of carbohydrates and only a few of them can be considered healthy carbohydrates from whole grains, starchy vegetables, beans, legumes, and fruits. Over time a high carbohydrate intake increases the risk of obesity, Type 2 Diabetes, and high triglycerides. However, other factors to consider in these health risks are genetics, blood sugar control, and physical activity level. Moderation, not elimination, is the key.

Keep in mind, too, any eating plan that severely restricts nutrients or foods can trigger constant thoughts and cravings for those foods, thereby upsetting internal cues of hunger and satiety. At its worst, restriction can lead to bingeing. When choosing a diet, analyze what works best for you. Is it to be no pasta ever or a sensible-sized portion when you are in the mood?

Worth A Try: Eating protein and fat satisfies hunger while you reduce calories from carbohydrates. Include whole grains, whole fruit, and vegetables in your carbohydrate allowance for optimal health.

Pass It By: The health benefits derived from the Atkins Diet, such as the improvement in metabolic syndrome, diabetes, and heart disease are nothing special to this diet and are common to many weight-loss diets. Acute carbohydrate restriction is difficult and unhealthy to sustain long-term and can cause severe and unhealthy side effects and nutrient deficiencies.

Wheat Belly And The Grain Brain Diet

Wheat Belly, the diet that cardiologist Dr. William Davis outlined in his book, became a sensation in its first month of publication.[10] In it, Dr. Davis contends that wheat consumption is to blame for obesity in the U.S. While he makes some solid points backed by scientific evidence, there are also false assertions and claims not backed by research, and statements that have been proven false leading readers to make unhealthy choices.

Davis' main argument, based on his use of comparisons to the weight of the U.S. population in the 1950's, links eating wheat to weight gain. While it is true that Americans were less likely to suffer from being overweight and obese in the middle of the last century, it takes more than just eating wheat to get that way.

I do agree with him on one thing and that is the damaging effects of refined grains, including wheat, because it is the type of carbohydrates that makes the biggest impact. Consumption of too many simple, processed carbohydrates, including wheat, leads to weight gain, what Davis calls wheat belly, the weight that accumulates around the mid-section of the torso. But, in general, it is common to notice belly fat with any type of weight gain. Eating whole grains, on the other hand, has been shown to promote weight maintenance, weight loss, lower body mass index, and reduced risk of obesity.[11] The merits of following the recommendations of the Wheat Belly Diet, such as the positive effects on blood sugars and liver issues, may simply be the result of losing weight.

The Wheat Belly Diet does emphasize eating vegetables, healthy fats from nuts, seeds and avocadoes, organic meats, eggs, and poultry— and it deserves kudos for that. Not so healthy is the diet's encouragement to eat lots of cheese and use sugar substitutes like Splenda, which can increase the risk of obesity.

Dr. David Perlmutter's book, *Grain Brain*, prescribes a diet similar to Wheat Belly.[12] Dr. Perlmutter makes some interesting points, the main one being that the wheat of today bears little resemblance to the wheat our ancestors enjoyed, or even the wheat grown half century ago. Many experts agree with Perlmutter that modern wheat may be difficult to digest and even cause other health issues. It's highly possible that wheat products today contain more gluten and that may explain the rise in gluten intolerance.

To illustrate the connection between wheat and weight, we need to look at the research conducted by Dr. Christine Zioudrou at the National Institutes of Health. Dr. Zioudrou discovered that wheat caused a drug-like state in mice and, among other things, also increased appetite. Could that drug-like state also be responsible for causing carb withdrawal? Self-proclaimed carboholics are nodding everywhere. It is also possible that modern wheat upsets the natural bacterial balance in the gut (referred to as the gut microbiome, discussed in depth in chapter 6) which has been shown to contribute to weight gain.

Dr. Perlmutter is correct in pointing out that we should not blame gluten as the only culprit affecting health. Indeed, all diets high in pro-inflammatory foods like sugar, beef, unhealthy fats, and environmental chemicals, also play a part in weight gain.

Dr. Perlmutter's Grain Brain diet claims that eating fat does not produce body fat and he recommends replacing calories from carbohydrates with foods high in fat. And that is cause for concern because, truth be told, dietary fat turns into body fat very easily with little or no thermogenesis (the calories expended when the body converts carbohydrates or protein to body fat). Dr. Perlmutter recommends eating 60-80 grams of carbohydrates a day, considered a severe restriction. The lack of vitamins, minerals and antioxidants in this eating style can contribute to a myriad of health issues. We have scientific evidence that proves whole grains make up an essential part of a healthy diet, but that grain does not have to be limited to wheat.

Dr. Perlmutter and I agree on the importance of including protein as part of a healthy breakfast. A morning meal with protein has the benefit of increasing satiety, controlling hunger, increasing metabolism, banishing carb cravings, and boosting energy levels. Because protein is best utilized by the body when it is spread out among several meals, it makes sense to start eating it at the first meal of the day.

Focus on eating lean protein: fish, eggs, low-sodium cottage cheese or low-fat Greek yogurt. In addition, protein powders like pea or hemp, popular plant-based alternatives, are easily incorporated into smoothies, oatmeal, and other grain and seed-based breakfast menus.

Is This Diet For You?

Worth A Try: Eliminating foods made from processed wheat including snack foods, breads and cereals is a diet strategy with great potential to flatten the belly. The emphasis on adequate lean protein intake will decrease hunger without adding the calories and unhealthy fats derived from high-fat meats. Like many other diets, reducing calories by removing wheat and other off-limit foods, generally leads to weight loss.

Pass It By: Extremely low carbohydrate diets are a quick fix, not a long-term solution. Severe carbohydrate restriction is not for anyone with diabetes or other blood sugar issues, or for pregnant or breastfeeding women. A registered dietitian nutritionist or your primary care physician can recommend the carbohydrate intake appropriate for you.

Gluten-Free Diet

This type of weight loss intervention arose because the proponents of wheat-free diets love to claim that everyone has a gluten sensitivity and that gluten causes a reaction in all humans. There is no scientific research to support this claim. Granted, there are extreme cases where gluten causes a profound change in the lining of the small intestine, where food is digested, but this is the result of Celiac disease, an auto-immune response where the body is attacking itself. The only treatment for Celiac disease is a complete life-long elimination of all wheat, barley, rye, and any foods that are contaminated by them. However, it is also true that some people are gluten sensitive or gluten intolerant and unaware. In these cases, gluten can be responsible for or can exacerbate health issues. For individuals with gluten issues, consuming gluten may change the amount of inflammation in the body, contributing to weight gain, but gluten-free diets themselves do not lead to weight loss. Other people who may find going gluten-free advantageous are those with inflammatory bowel disease, irritable bowel disease, and auto-immune health issues like thyroid disease. However, studies show evidence that people without gluten sensitivities or intolerances, and who eat whole grains, have lower inflammation in the body, reducing their risk of weight issues. This means that those without a gluten intolerance or Celiac Disease do not have to eliminate gluten from their diet in order to lose weight. It is imperative that you see a doctor to rule out the possibility of Celiac Disease before considering a gluten-free diet. In reality, only about 1% of the population has Celiac Disease and perhaps 10% or less have a gluten sensitivity. As for the rest, their bodies may be revolting from overconsumption of gluten and not from a problem with the gluten itself.

There is also the fact that weight loss and improved health by eliminating wheat may not be attributable to gluten at all, but possibly yet another compound present in the food that is harmful to some individuals. Remember too that gluten-free foods are not carbohydrate free. This is because the gluten is replaced with other carbohydrates, such as gluten-free flour, tapioca starch, rice starch, and corn starch, all of which your body uses as it does any other carbohydrate-containing food. Be careful: gluten-free carbohydrates still add calories sufficient enough to prevent weight loss.

The popularity of gluten-free diets has skyrocketed to a multi-billion-dollar industry globally. Gluten diets have been touted by some as a weight-loss plan and followed by others as healthy eating. This combination makes going gluten-free the *of-the-moment* trend causing an explosion in sales of gluten-free foods. According to a survey by Statista, 12% of gluten-free followers were looking toward healthier eating while 7% were using gluten free as a weight loss diet, making it all the more ironic that the greatest growth in production of gluten-free foods has been in breads, cookies, and snack foods. To a much lesser degree, the trendy gluten-free diet is fueled by an increase in the number of individuals diagnosed with Celiac Disease or gluten sensitivity, and to a greater degree by what the public perceives as a healthy diet with media marketing and celebrity endorsements fueling the flames.

How did gluten get its bad reputation? Gluten is a protein found in wheat, barley, and rye. At one time, oats were also on that list, but we now know that oats do not contain gluten unless they are contaminated by machinery that also processes wheat. It is also interesting to point out that removing the grains—wheat, barley, and rye—does not eliminate all gluten from the diet since gluten is also used in thickeners, binders, food coloring, and flavorings. It is also added to food in the form of maltodextrin, modified corn starch and other substances commonly found in ingredient lists. Many people are unaware of this, including those with Celiac or a gluten intolerance for whom removing all the gluten from their diet is imperative. For those who do not remove all traces of gluten from the diet but still feel better or lose weight, it's probably not a gluten intolerance but the elimination of an overload of processed foods and convenience foods. They are most likely feeling better because they are eating fewer carbohydrates over-all and more vegetables and fruits. Also, reducing intake of processed and convenience foods means consuming fewer toxins and chemicals that are pervasive in the typical American diet.

It is also common for those who assume that gluten-free is healthier and/or lower in carbohydrates to consume large amounts of gluten-free pretzels, cereals, and crackers. Wrong! Those foods are just as processed and ill-advised as their gluten-containing counterparts. Using a gluten-free diet for weight loss can, instead, lead to weight gain. Often, to make a gluten-free food taste good and have an appealing texture, high amounts of fat and sugar are added to gluten free flours, making them higher in calories per serving as compared to their mainstream counterparts. This means that in order to lose weight on a gluten-free diet, it's important to focus on portion controlled vegetables, fruits, high fiber whole grains, lean meats, healthy fats, lean proteins, and minimally processed foods and to avoid added fats and sugars, the same recommendations common to all successful weight loss programs.

What The Experts Say

Along with gluten, this diet also eliminates many vitamins and minerals especially the B vitamins and iron. Even though the body doesn't miss gluten, it will suffer from the loss of those nutrients in addition to the fiber wheat, barley, and rye add to the diet.[13]

When considering a gluten-free diet, it is important to consult a physician first because gastro-intestinal symptoms need to be addressed to rule out Celiac disease. For the tests to be accurate, you must be consuming gluten when the tests are conducted.[14]

There are also blood tests that have proven fully accurate in helping identify non-celiac gluten sensitivity. If you get a green light from your doctor and want to follow a gluten-free diet, there are a few things to consider…

What is known about non-Celiac gluten sensitivity:

- Many anecdotal accounts, but not much scientific study conclusions, about gluten-free diets lessening symptoms for irritable bowel syndrome, autism spectrum disorders, eczema, psoriasis, constipation, diarrhea, and bloating can be found.

- Removing gluten from the diet completely, after Celiac is ruled out, helps identify gluten sensitivity.

- Gluten-free foods are up to 242% more expensive than their regularly manufactured counterparts.

- When gluten is removed from foods, manufacturers routinely add fat and sugar to replace the texture qualities.

- Processed gluten-free foods are lower in vitamins, minerals, and fiber.

- When following a gluten-free diet, always consult a registered dietitian nutritionist, to keep the diet nutritious and sustainable.

Is This Diet For You?

Worth A Try: A Gluten-free diet may remove a food sensitivity that could potentially be the source of intestinal discomfort, fatigue, and brain fog. Just feeling better can help you become more motivated to make the diet and lifestyle changes that lead to weight loss. Eating more foods that are naturally gluten-free, like lean proteins, vegetables, and fruits, is a lower carb approach, can reduce calorie intake and, as a weight loss strategy, points to greater success.

Pass It By: Going gluten-free is unlikely to lead to weight loss success. If you choose a Gluten-free diet, don't rely on convenience foods and packaged items, which are generally higher in calories than their conventional counterparts. Also, be prepared to spend more at the supermarket.

Ketogenic Diet

The Ketogenic diet is another low carbohydrate diet that is much stricter than Atkins. A true Ketogenic diet, as developed by the medical community, is distinctly different from other low carb diets in that protein intake also stays low and the focus is on high fat that averages 75-90% of total daily calories and by limiting daily carbohydrate intake to 20 grams. Most people who claim to follow a Ketogenic diet are, in fact, on a modified Atkins diet with the calories from both protein and fat making up for the lack of carbohydrates. The current popular version of the Keto diet is similar to the Atkins Diet with a daily carb limit set at 50 grams (less than a typical breakfast muffin). Without strict adherence to guidelines there is a wide variation in weight loss results. Also, the harsh reality is only 45% of Keto diet followers are able to stick with it long enough to see results.[15]

How It Works

I must emphasize the importance of medical supervision for anyone on a Ketogenic diet plan because of extreme carbohydrate restriction.

A Ketogenic diet severely restricts carbohydrate consumption, causing the body to switch from carbohydrates to fats as fuel. Most of this fat comes from food but some comes from body fat and this is intentional but can cause problems. When the body uses fat as fuel, it produces ketones which are acid by-products of this process. Having high levels of ketones in the blood and urine is referred to as being in the state of ketosis and this state is reached in as long as one to two weeks on a low carbohydrate, low protein, high-fat diet. Because the body has the ability to convert proteins to carbohydrates, eating too much protein prevents ketosis and the utilization of body fat for fuel. Any diversion from the high-fat/very low-carb diet, no matter how small or temporary, and the state of ketosis is halted. That means no splurging whatsoever.

The Ketogenic diet consists of eating fat from animal proteins, whole eggs, most cheeses, butter, cream, mayonnaise, nuts, seeds, coconut and other oils. Forbidden foods include starchy vegetables (peas, corn, potatoes, beans, legumes), milk/yogurt, fruits, grains (bread, potato, cereal, pasta, rice), all sweeteners and sweets (pastries, cookies, cakes, ice cream, candy), peppers, carrots, beets and onions.

Because food choices are limited, this diet often becomes boring as textures and flavors are limited too. This makes the Keto diet hard to sustain over the long haul due to the strict rules and the repetitive menus of meat, fish, chicken, eggs, and a lot of greens. One Ketogenic follower described her breakfast as eggs with lots of butter, bacon, and avocado. Another follower ate eggs, cheese, spinach, and tomato. A typical lunch consists of chicken and 5 cups of salad greens or a beef stir fry made with coconut oil, and vegetables. Dinner may be chicken soup or a plate of pork, broccoli, and salad. Other meals may consist of an almond milk peanut butter smoothie, handful of nuts, celery sticks, guacamole and salsa, romaine lettuce wraps of ham and cheese. Snacks include olives, almonds, cheese, peanut butter, and hard-boiled eggs with mayo. Many foods are prepared using butter and coconut milk (in fact, butter and mayo are most often used in the menus which, at the present time, is not considered to be heart healthy).

The original Ketogenic diet was developed by medical experts almost 100 years ago but today's Keto diet, promoted for weight loss, is different. In the original diet, 75-90% of daily calories came from fat, 10-25% from protein and carbohydrates combined. Today's version has a higher protein model of 60% of calories from fat and 35% of calories from protein. In both cases, carbohydrates are limited to 5% of total calories. The higher protein option may be healthier because it helps you maintain muscle mass while losing body fat. The downside is that it may make it more difficult to stay in ketosis and, therefore, less effective.

The Ketogenic Mediterranean Diet is another alternative version of this diet and is more liberal in its fat, protein, and carbohydrate ratios and supports eating healthy polyunsaturated and monounsaturated fats and lean proteins. This alternative is less restrictive and may be easier to follow.

Ketogenic diets provide a consistent energy source by constantly breaking down body fat for fuel while providing satiating high-fat meals that can result in reduced hunger and cravings, thereby lowering total daily calories resulting in weight loss. Keep in mind, though, weight is lost only if the number of calories burned remains greater than the calories consumed. So, there is a calorie restriction component to this diet in addition to the carbohydrate restriction that contributes to the significant weight loss touted in using this method.

What The Experts Say

The Ketogenic diet has been used for almost one hundred years by physicians to treat epilepsy, seizure disorders, and cancer. Current research has shown promising results using this diet to manage other health issues, including migraines, depression, diabetes, and Alzheimer's. Only lately has the Ketogenic diet been adopted for weight loss, mostly without the necessary medical supervision. It's also a hot trend with a growing number of bloggers and cookbook authors. The typical fad version allows 20-50 grams of carbohydrates a day, that's 5-10% of total calorie intake. Compare that to the typical American diet, which includes 50-65% of calories from carbohydrates. Many dieters do not reach ketosis because the low amount of carbohydrates necessary to do so is unattainable. About 20% of calories comes from protein, which is still adequate for most people to maintain healthy bodily functions. The key nutrient is dietary fat, which makes up about 75% of daily calories.

There are no long-term studies on using a Ketogenic diet for weight loss, and only a few minor short-term studies One significant finding from a review of these studies highlights the noticeable decrease in appetite. These studies suggest a reduced appetite may be due either to the satiating effect of the fat and protein or the presence of ketones in the blood. It is also possible the loss of appetite comes from a loss of interest in food since the choices are so limited. Research also suggests that high-fat diets reduce appetite hormone levels, which in turn decrease appetite and calorie intake. Researchers also questioned whether there is a need for such a drastic reduction in carbohydrates to experience a reduction in appetite. They suggested similar benefits could be had by limiting carbs to 50 grams per day instead of 20 grams as instructed by the Ketogenic diet. Unfortunately, within two weeks of going off this type of diet, many subjects reported their hunger and cravings were even higher than before going on the diet.

Medical experts are concerned most that the use of Ketogenic diets will lead to deficiencies in vital nutrients, including vitamins, minerals, and fiber. There is also concern that this eating plan will lead to imbalances in the gut, compromising digestive health. Some studies show Keto improves LDL (bad) cholesterol levels while others warn that this diet is linked to elevated LDL cholesterol and clogged blood vessels. Without long-term studies, the Keto diet remains questionable in regard to heart health.

Is This Diet For You?

A Ketogenic diet may be an effective way of losing weight because eating fat helps you feel full, a perk when dieting. Fat also provides the taste and texture in food that we all enjoy. The loss of appetite that ketosis causes, along with the nausea, light-headedness, and fatigue, also reduces intake and the desire to eat. It is this loss of appetite that makes it possible for the body to starve without feeling hungry. The increased protein intake may also be effective at reducing appetite by increasing feelings of satiety. What's more, burning body fat for fuel reduces fat stores and increases metabolic rate.

Along with low energy, light-headedness and nausea, many users of this diet also report constipation, and headaches at first, referred to as keto flu, but many of these side effects resolve once the body adapts. The Ketogenic diet can also have more lasting consequences, including increased incidence of kidney stones and nutrient deficiencies. Because this diet is so restrictive, taking vitamins and mineral supplements is recommended. Other negative reactions are continued fatigue, dizziness, low blood sugar, muscle cramps, dry mouth, bad breath, excessive urination, and sleep disturbances. Many of these side effects are caused by extreme water loss and can be countered by increasing water intake and replacing electrolytes (not with Gatorade or other sports drinks that are high in hidden carbs). Boost electrolytes by regularly incorporating avocado, sea salt, leafy greens, and lemons into meals. Exercise performance may also be compromised. With fuel from carbs in short supply (the body requires less oxygen to burn carbs than fat for energy)…any high intensity demand on the body from running sprints to weightlifting to climbing stairs may be difficult. There is some concern about the loss of muscle mass. To reduce the risk, adequate protein, and exercise, especially weight training, is advised.

Hormone and genetic differences cause some users to lose a lot of weight while others experience minimal weight loss (8-10 lbs. in 4 weeks is a reasonable expectation). Also present here, as in all highly restrictive eating plans, is the common dieting danger of long-term food restrictions. These restrictions often lead to strong cravings for forbidden foods, especially sugar, as well as the tendency to overeat. Remember, one splurge and ketosis ends, and it's back to the severe restrictions taking up to two weeks to get back into ketosis. The return to eating carbohydrates often causes the regain of lost weight unless a maintenance plan is in place.

Individual studies report greater weight loss on a Ketogenic diet when compared to other low carb diets. The current version of the Keto diet is most popular because of quick weight loss, often 5-15 pounds in a few weeks. However, combining data from several studies showed that 13 trials totaling 1,400 participants revealed those on the Ketogenic diet lost only an average of an extra two pounds after one year, compared to a low-fat or other conventional diet, with **no difference** in weight loss after two years. Yikes! All that restriction for 0-2 pounds. The reasons may be because fat loss slows as the body breaks down muscle for energy, or the monotony of the food choices and/or the elimination of food groups translates more to less eating and not the avoidance of carbohydrates.[16]

Using the ketogenic method produces immediate weight loss because of the initial water losses. Rapid weight loss may continue, but results vary greatly. Again, there must be strict adherence to the carbohydrate restriction to sustain keto-adaptation and weight loss. In addition, this diet requires that urine be monitored daily with test strips used first thing in the morning to confirm the presence of ketones indicating the body is in the state of ketosis.

This is not a weight-loss method widely recommended by the medical community. If you are contemplating a Ketogenic diet for weight loss, it is important to first consult with your doctor. You will also need guidance in meal options because of the lack of carbohydrates and excess fat in allowable foods. Eliminating grains, fruits, vegetables, beans, and legumes increases risk of deficiencies in calcium, Vitamin D, magnesium, iron, selenium, and essential fatty acids.

The Ketogenic diet also poses challenges to vegetarians and vegans who may find it necessary to include dairy and eggs for adequate protein because the carbohydrate content of plant-based proteins may hamper reaching ketosis. The Ketogenic diet is also risky for those with a history of kidney stones, high cholesterol, or are concerned about prostate or kidney cancer. A registered dietitian nutritionist can provide guidance needed to lose weight while maintaining good health. Be aware that transitioning from Keto must be gradual as the Ketogenic diet reduces the body's ability to metabolize carbohydrates.

Worth A Try: If you prefer knowing exactly which foods can be eaten at will and which must be avoided, as opposed to counting grams or measuring portion sizes, this may be an option for you. Fats add texture to foods and help you feel full longer, which may make it easier to stick with this diet with a good chance you will not go hungry while losing weight. The initial quick weight loss might jump-start your efforts or even increase your motivation to choose or transition to another method.

Pass It By: Several medical conditions make the Ketogenic diet downright dangerous. For example, do not even consider the Ketogenic diet if you are pregnant or breast-feeding, or have a genetic predisposition to high cholesterol. Then there is the constipation issue as well as deficiencies in calcium, vitamin D, vitamin C, and some B vitamins. Less serious cons include boredom from the short list of allowed foods and the challenge to your social life. This diet is tough to follow especially if you are a social eater. Keto diets require advance meal-planning, a well-equipped kitchen, and no cheating on weekends (which many dieters do). This diet is so hard to sustain that few are truly able to follow it long enough to see lasting results.

Again, please, please, please consult a physician before looking into this diet any further.

Volumetrics

Volumetrics was developed by Barbara Rolls, Ph.D., professor of nutritional sciences and obesity researcher at Penn State University. The Volumetrics eating plan is based on studies conducted in research laboratories regarding portion size, fat content, and calorie density. This plan is effective, safe, and maintainable long-term.

How It Works

The outstanding feature of this diet is not being hungry because you will be eating more food with fewer calories. This is possible by consuming foods with high water content that lowers calorie density to allow you to enjoy larger portions. Filling up on low-calorie, high water and high fiber foods, namely fruits, vegetables, soups and stews translates into losing weight while eating more. Let me say it again to be sure you got it right. You can eat more on this plan than you are eating today and still lose weight![17]

On Volumetrics, you don't have to measure food or count calories, but you do need to be aware of portion sizes. This method of weight loss relies on hunger control. We are born with internal cues that tell us when it's time to eat and when it's time to stop. Just try to over feed a baby. Babies push food away, turn their heads, or spit it out when full. But babies turn into adults who eventually learn they don't need to be hungry in order to eat. We eat because food tastes good.

And we don't always listen to our gut when it tells us to stop eating. With practice you can retrain yourself to be aware of the moment in a meal when you have had enough. Hunger control also includes eating when you are hungry because waiting until you are ravenous leads to overeating. We all know how hard it is to control portion sizes when we are so hungry we shovel in the food to fill the nagging hole in our gut. Serial dieters actually lose the ability to recognize hunger cues due to and contributing to their restrictive and overeating behaviors. When this happens, those natural signs of hunger and fullness must be relearned and practiced in order to again become aware of what the body is trying to tell you. If this is happening to you, regularly ask yourself, "Am I hungry?" because eating when you are mild to moderately hungry is the best way to control portion sizes. Checking in while you are eating will help you determine when you have had enough.

Volumetrics works because it fills your plate with fruits and vegetables, the least calorie-dense foods, while judiciously including vegetable oils, nuts, and nut butters, translating to fewer calories. This diet is easy to maintain because it allows many more foods, and some may surprise you. You can enjoy oatmeal made with water, soups, sweet and white potatoes, black beans, white rice, and spaghetti cooked in water, skinless turkey breast, extra lean ham, low-fat yogurt, some whole grain cereals with low-fat milk and certain fish. Considering that fats have more than twice the number of calories compared to carbohydrates or proteins, portions of high-fat foods are smaller. Low-fat foods mean bigger portions for the same number of calories. But don't worry about loss of flavor. Volumetrics shares lots of tips on cooking methods and other ways to replace the flavor that fats provide.

What this plan excels at is that it includes all foods. Its focus is on what <u>can</u> be eaten not what can't be eaten. It stresses creating balanced meals and ways to relearn hunger and fullness cues to help with portion control. Volumetrics promotes ways to develop a satisfying relationship with food that will last a lifetime to keep the weight off.

Volumetrics instructs you to choose most foods from the very-low-density and low-density groups, to carefully control portions of foods in the medium-density group, and eat a minimal amount from the high-density category. This combination keeps you satisfied and limits foods that may trigger overindulging. Foods that fall in the categories of very-low-density and low-density are most fruits and vegetables, low-fat yogurt, soups, and some fish, while meats, cheeses, French fries and ice cream would be deemed medium-density foods. Cookies, crackers, chips, nuts, butter and oil are highly calorie dense.

What The Experts Say

Volumetrics was developed by an expert, based on twenty-five years in the field of nutrition and weight management. Since its publication in 2005, Volumetrics has led the pack in effective weight loss without the drudgery of a typical weight loss diet. In fact, 13 studies concluded there is a connection between low calorie density foods and weight loss.[18] All studies comparing the use of low calorie-dense foods to other diet modalities found eating low caloriedense foods led to greater weight loss.[19][20][21][22] Remarkably, every subject in the Volumetrics studies lost weight without restrictions in calories, carbohydrates or fats per se. Choosing low calorie-dense foods led to eating more vegetables and fruits crowding out the high calorie foods with hidden fats and carbs, typically filling the plate. Volumetrics stresses food choices over calorie count or carbohydrate content.

Is This Diet For You?

Where most diets are restrictive and leave you walking around feeling hungry, Volumetrics keeps you satisfied and does not eliminate any foods that may trigger overindulging. Check out visuals online, which are immensely helpful in understanding calorie density. For example, see how a quarter cup of nuts compares with 25 cups of raw spinach, both providing approximately 175 calories.[24]

The Volumetrics diet books include recipes to help with meal planning and food shopping. Because this diet does not eliminate or restrict any food groups, it has a leg up over the competition because it promotes healthy eating. You are free to enjoy favorite foods with only a modification in serving size or perhaps a change of toppings or dips. It also fits in with any lifestyle or dietary preference, including gluten-free, vegetarian/vegan, kosher, and halal. An added bonus, Volumetrics also allows alcohol in moderation.

Worth A Try: Eating low-calorie dense foods allows you to consume fewer calories in a higher volume of food so you feel fuller. Fruits and vegetables are high in fiber, which promotes that feeling of fullness while reducing calorie intake. Eating satisfying meals also means needing smaller or fewer snacks between meals, eliminating additional calories. Because many low calorie-dense foods are high in nutrient content, there is little risk of nutrient deficiencies. The protein-rich foods also help satisfy hunger and preserve muscle while losing body fat.

Pass It By: If your food preferences make eating fruits and vegetables challenging, this is not a diet you can adhere to. This plan also encourages home-prepared meals, so if you do not have access to a kitchen or you don't like to cook, this diet is not for you.

Paleo Diet

Some people claim that today's problem with weight and health is because our diets have changed so drastically over thousands of years of human evolution. The Paleo Diet, aka Caveman Diet, aka Hunter-Gatherer Diet, encourages eating as our ancestors did 10,000 years ago, which means, according to Paleo enthusiasts, not eating grains, beans, legumes, or dairy. Proponents of "stone-age" eating blame the adding of grains, legumes, and dairy to our diet after the agricultural revolution for today's rise in obesity, diabetes, and heart disease.

How It Works

The Paleo Diet focuses on foods that were either hunted or gathered. This means meat, poultry, fish, fruits, vegetables, avocado, nuts, seeds, and plant-based oils, including olive, walnut, and coconut. Encouraging consumption of more vegetables and fruits and elimination of sugar and sodium are always heathy food habits to practice. Those healthy eating habits, along with a higher percentage of calories from protein, are why paleo eating can lead to weight loss.

The following is a sample weight-loss meal plan for one day, from The Paleo Solution by Robb Wolf. [24]

Breakfast: Shrimp scramble with basil and steamed spinach. ¼ cup blueberries. Espresso

Lunch: Chicken salad with red onions, romaine lettuce, artichoke hearts and mixed bell peppers. Dressing: Lemon/olive oil with a hint of garlic. Green tea with lemon.

Snack: Grilled shrimp & veggies with a handful of macadamias.

Dinner: Baked pork loin with ginger cabbage and olive oil. Dessert: shaved almonds over 1/4 cup mixed berries.

What The Experts Say

The ideas behind the Paleo Diet are not supported by anthropologists (If this topic interests you, look up the Ted Talk by Christina

Warinner).[25] Humans have big molars for mashing (think vegetarian) and only a few sharp incisors for tearing and shredding, which does not support the Paleo Diet practice of high animal protein intake. Paleolithic people ate lean, small animals, not large domesticated ones like cows. We also know that eating too much protein and fat and not enough carbohydrates and dairy (another paleo no-no) increases risks of nutrient deficiencies.

The Paleo Diet eliminates grains and legumes, which also means eliminating fiber. Our ancestors were gatherers who ate a diverse variety of plant food, so their diet was undoubtedly very high in fiber, possibly 100 grams a day, as compared to today's average of 15 grams of fiber per day. The claim that Paleolithic people did not eat grains has also been refuted by archeological evidence of 10,000-year-old stones used for grinding grains and seeds.

On the other hand, there are also ancient foods that are no longer modern diet staples. This begs the question, is the current obesity problem caused by the foods added to our diet by the agricultural revolution or because we eat too much processed foods? And about the high vegetable intake of those hunter-gatherers of old, Centers for Disease Control and Prevention reports that today only one in ten Americans eats the daily recommended amount of fruits and vegetables.[26]

Another problem with the Paleo Diet rationale is that ancient people ate a diverse diet. In truth, hunter-gatherer diets varied widely depending on which plants were in season and what animals were available. For instance, during dry seasons, early humans relied on meats, but the wet seasons brought an abundance of plants, especially berries. Vegetables, fruits, nuts, and oils were available in all seasons.

There is also the larger mystery that remains of knowing exactly what people really ate back then. We also don't know on which continent this diet is based. Back then, people ate what was around them and they migrated from place to place with the changing of the seasons to find better food supplies.

Paleo-archeologist Peter Ungar reported in *Scientific American* that the current fad diet does not resemble what paleolithic humans ate. He also noted that cereal grains were used by some cultures and that ancient diets varied around the world based on climate and what was available. Ungar's findings support dietary flexibility, a definite endorsement to eating seasonally and locally, and maybe an explanation as to why we can't all manage our weight in the same way.[27]

Proponents of the Paleo Diet contend that we carry the same genes as our ancestors of 10,000 years ago when, in fact, evolutionary biologists have found evidence to the contrary. Yes, humans evolved from hunter-gatherers to farmers, but our genes evolved, too. Modern humans have some genes ancient humans lacked. Gene mutations arose from an agriculturally based diet and the domestication of cows, allowing us the ability to digest and absorb nutrients from grains, milk, and cheeses. Some genes adapted to these modern changes in the food supply, but most did not. The availability of modern foods is not solely responsible for weight problems and poor health, but unhealthy diet practices in the most recent hundred years *is*, as we now consume more processed grains, rather than whole, and large quantities of cheese. Common sense tells us that it's not the inability to digest grains and dairy that is causing today's health and weight issues…it's because we eat too much of them.

Is This Diet For You?

The Paleo Diet may be an unhealthy choice as it eliminates entire food groups, reducing consumption of the valuable nutrients found in those foods. For example, the Paleo Diet eliminates whole grains with the key nutrients B vitamins, magnesium, and fiber, and dairy foods providing the highest amount of calcium for those of us who live in the United States, which is important to bone health. Newer studies point to eating calcium-rich foods as leading to higher body fat loss. The lowest calcium consumers in these studies had the most belly fat. Consider that it is not our diet but the composition of the grains that has changed. Industrialization of farming has altered the grains we eat. The unhealthy influences of those grains are real. But remember, not all of them are manufactured with unhealthy practices. So instead of eliminating all of them from your diet, a better approach would be to eat foods that are less processed to avoid any altered by science, including GMOs, preservatives, additives, and pesticides.

Eliminating dairy and grains may help heal the gut in people with digestive disorders and improve gut health. Resolving digestive issues too may also contribute to successful weight loss. Eliminating grains and dairy short-term should have little impact on overall health. That said, a nutrition assessment by a registered dietitian nutritionist can determine what, if any, nutrients are lacking in any diet. Alternative sources of those nutrients and proper meal planning can make up for gaps caused by the restrictions of this diet.

The anthropological evidence points to eating regionally, seasonally, locally small portions, and adding tough woody produce (broccoli, artichoke, asparagus), and that's good (yes, folks, more reasons to eat those fruits and vegetables). We may not have access to wild game as our ancestors did, but you can instead choose wild-caught fish and grass-fed meat.

The elimination of beans on a weight loss diet is a contradiction to findings of a study of 21 food trials, which concluded that eating beans, chickpeas, and lentils (aka "pulses") helped dieters lose weight and prevented regaining it. Researchers also noted the full feeling that these high-fiber foods provided as the reason for weight-loss success. Beans have a low glycemic index, meaning that they are digested slowly with low effect on insulin levels as they provide protein without fat, a healthy substitute for animal protein.[28]

Menopause introduces women to changes in weight and shifts in body fat. Of great concern is the thickening of the waist, more abdominal fat, and rising lipid levels. For post-menopausal women on the Paleo Diet, studies show significantly more body fat loss at 6 months when compared to less restrictive diets. But after two years following the same diets, one diet showed no advantage over the other in total body fat loss. It is worth noting, though, that the decrease in waist circumference and triglyceride levels was distinctively greater for women on the Paleo Diet. These results are promising but more studies need to be done to see if men experience the same benefits. Also important is that there are many variations of the Paleo Diet that may not yield identical results to the ones used in the studies.[29]

The Pros of the Paleo diet:
- Diversity, creating a varied diet

- Limited processed foods, especially corn, soy, wheat, and oils

- Promotes eating fresh foods that are naturally preserved by drying, salting, smoking, and pickling to inhibit bacterial growth with no chemical additives or preservatives that may affect good bacteria in the gut and lead to obesity

- Recommends eating whole foods high in fiber to help satiety, blood sugar control, cholesterol levels, and feed healthy bacteria

Worth A Try: The Paleo diet may be a good strategy for dieters who need a "good foods, bad foods" list to focus on what to eat instead of what not to eat. If you consume too much sugar and refined carbohydrates, this diet also helps to avoid over-processed and packaged foods. Vegetables and fruits are included at every meal and help to form life-long healthy eating habits and curtail dependence on grain-based food products.

Pass It By: Eating dairy-free and gluten-free can lead to nutrient deficits, including calcium, iron, fiber, and B vitamins. If your choice of vegetables and fruits is limited, or if produce is unavailable, there won't be enough variety on this plan and boredom and deprivation will set in rapidly. The Paleo Diet is hard on the wallet and won't work for anyone on a food budget.

Intermittent Fasting (IF)

Intermittent fasts regulate the time frame in which you allow yourself to eat, which may help lead to easier or greater success in weight loss.

Intermittent Fast eating patterns:
- Limiting eating to the same 6-12 hours daily

- Alternating patterns of under- and over-eating days

- 5 days of eating normally, 2 fasting days per week

- Random fast, aka meal skipping

- Having regular splurge days in the middle of a calorie-restricted diet

To be clear, fasting is, by definition, a willing abstention from all food, and often fluids, for a specified time period. Modified fasting, abstaining from food for a shortened time frame, is typically recommended by many of the fast-type diets.

Fasting can either be a change in lifestyle or a catalyst to shake free of old habits. Fasting may also provide perspective on eating habits, shine a light on unhealthy eating patterns, elevate mood and increase energy level. These outcomes can lead to a more positive attitude, which in turn leads to greater effort put into whatever method comes next. Fasting may be spiritual, leading to a focus on the mind-body connection much like yoga. The feeling of enlightenment, clarity and inner peace may help change one's relationship with food, making it possible to identify and change emotional eating. It can also alter a perceived dependence on sugar and processed foods and, after an extended period of time, eliminate food choices often referred to as cravings.[30]

How It Works

There are several popular forms of intermittent fasting.

The 5:2 diet calls for eating without restriction for 5 days followed by consuming a sparse 500-600 calories on 2 non-consecutive "fasting" days. Some variations allow only certain kinds of foods on "fasting" days. Some juice and liquid diets fall into this category.

Another type of IF, Alternate Day fasting, limits food to 500 calories every other day. "Feast" days allow you to eat whatever you want, often 1500-2000 calories. By alternating one feast day followed by one fast day, there are more fast days per week than prescribed in the 5:2 diet.

One more version of IF—Time-Restricted fasting—limits intake to 6-12 hours out of the day, abstaining from any intake for the remaining 12-18 hours of the day, and does not specify guidelines for amount or composition of food consumed.

What The Experts Say

5:2 Intermittent Fasting

There is growing evidence of more successful weight loss using intermittent fasting methods compared to the continuous calorie restriction of most dieting plans. In studies comparing intermittent fasting to continuous calorie restriction over 8-12 weeks, dieters in both groups lost 6-8% of body weight.[31] However, the success of the 5:2 IF method may be dependent on curbing calories on the 5 feast days and not eating whatever you want on non-fast days.[32]

Here is an interesting difference between the continuous calorie restriction method and the 5:2 method. With intermittent fasting, dieters were able to reduce their average daily calorie intake (the average of fast and feast days) by a total of 35-38%. Subjects following the continuous calorie restriction method reduced their average daily intake by only 18-23%. Also, a higher amount of body fat was lost with intermittent fasting, 90% fat 10% lean body mass (LBM). Using continuous calorie restriction, weight lost was 75% fat and 25% LBM. The same amount of weight was lost using both methods, however, more body fat was lost using IF.[33]

There is a compelling explanation for why intermittent fasting is an effective method of losing weight. Mark Mattson at the National Institute on Aging explains that for much of human existence, our bodies evolved to be accustomed to limited availability of food (think hunter-gatherer lifestyle of earlier societies). This led to our development of organ systems, liver, and muscles that easily store and retrieve carbohydrates for fuel, and fat that holds onto long-lasting energy reserves—important to sustain us when there was no access to food. So intermittent fasting closely resembles the feast-or-famine availability of food that our ancestors experienced, which influenced how our bodies used and stored food for energy. Having 24-hour access to food is just not in our DNA.

Alternate-Day IF

Intermittent fasting is not yet fully understood. So far, most information has been gleaned from studies using rodents as subjects and with few clinical trials on human subjects. One short-term study, reported May 2017, involved 100 participants following either an alternate-day fast diet or continuous calorie-restricted diet. Researchers found subjects on the alternate day fast ate more than they should have on fast days and less than advised on the feast days. Subjects on the continuous calorie restricted diet followed recommended daily calorie intake more precisely. This suggests that you may be more successful using an intermittent fasting method if you have specific calorie goals for both feast days and fast days.

Also, sticking to a fasting plan was harder to do with more dieters quitting the study than those in the continuous calorie restriction group. At the end of six months and after one year, weight loss was similar in the two groups, showing that the more effective diet is the one you can live with.

Longer two-year studies on overweight but not obese adults showed they could eat 12% fewer calories than normal for a 10% change in body weight, but were unsuccessful at cutting more calories than that. When asked to eat normally five days and restrict to 25% of normal on two days, the subjects lost the same amount of weight and more body fat. Similar results were found in a study involving obese men and women. The research thus far is cause for optimism.

Besides weight loss, Alternate-Day Intermittent Fasting can reduce insulin resistance, LDL-cholesterol and triglycerides, all metabolic markers important for optimal health.

Time Restricted Fasting

Time-restricted diets reduce the hours of the day when eating is allowed. This would be, for example, eating the last meal/snack of the day within a 6-10-hour window from the first food of the day. During the fasting period, usually a more than 12-hour stretch, the body relies on fat for energy, helping to use up stored body fat leading to weight loss. Eliminating even a few hours from a typical feeding pattern can trigger fat loss and lead to sustainable weight loss.

The OMAD (One Meal A Day) is the latest time-restricted fasting diet to hit the media. This is just another restrictive diet that causes health issues, brain fog, fatigue, and erratic blood sugars along with quick but unsustainable weight loss.

The Snake Diet, marketed by Cole Robinson, a fitness trainer with no known nutrition or medical credentials, also pops up in internet searches. Robinson's advice is rather alarming as it recommends to "fast as long as possible every day while still getting in all of the calories and macro/micronutrients your body needs." He claims that fasting time counts, and for optimal weight loss all food should be consumed within one to two hours (a video online suggests 30 seconds). The body is unable to get what nutrients it needs to preserve good health in that short period of time. This diet will most certainly cause headaches, low energy, and bad moods. The only reason for including this preposterous idea is to highlight how important it is to choose a *healthy* fasting plan presented by a reputable source.

The pairing of time-restricted fasting with other diets is also popular. Intermittent fasting is easily paired with other diets because it is a meal pattern and not a diet prescription. Simply follow the guidelines of a chosen diet within a specific window of time, typically eight hours. For example, a popular combination is combining Keto with fasting 16 hours a day to reach ketosis quicker, but look out, you also get double the side effects.

Besides weight loss, research on time-restricted fasting (keeping meals and snacks within a healthy 8-10-hour window) shows it can result in lower blood pressure, cholesterol, and triglycerides as well as increased insulin sensitivity, reduced cancer risk and inflammation.[34]

A Fast-Mimicking Diet (FMD), currently under investigation, prescribing low calories, sugars, and protein but high unsaturated fat intake for five consecutive days a month, reduces inflammation and aging, and age-related diseases. Additional good news is that this Fast-Mimicking Diet is showing promise in the treatment of inflammatory bowel disease.[35] A gastroenterologist can determine if FMD is appropriate and provide specific guidelines for effectiveness.[36]

Harnessing Your Circadian Rhythm

Humans have an internal biological clock, a natural 24-hour cycle known as circadian rhythm. Circadian rhythms create predictable changes in bodily functions and behaviors. The Circadian rhythm is affected by light, dark, temperature, time zones, and sleep patterns. Disruptions in circadian rhythm affect weight. Skipping meals, sleep deprivation, a sedentary lifestyle, and random food consumption also affect this internal clock, which in turn affects weight, and not in a good way. Getting enough sleep, 7-9 hours every night, without disruption, and consistently going to bed and rising at the same time of day, supports hormones that regulate stress, appetite, and food choices including total sugar intake and cravings for salty or sweet foods.[37] Poor quantity and quality of sleep makes you hungrier and leads to increased eating between meals, often high carbohydrate foods to comfort food cravings. How much hungrier, you may ask? Almost 400 additional calories hungry.[38] An excellent example of this concerns night shift workers, who researchers found have a high percentage of obesity and other health issues. The key to these findings is the effect of the lifestyle on their metabolism, which translates into the importance of timing meals, but it is your internal clock you should be following and not the one on your computer screen. The benefit to choosing an 8 to 12-hour window for eating between sun-up and sundown is that consuming 3 meals within 8 hours reduces the need to snack between meals, leading to decreased calorie intake. It also eliminates high calorie eating at night when physical activity and, therefore, calorie needs, are low. Carbohydrates should be consumed mostly in the morning and early afternoon when metabolism is at its highest.

Studies by Mark Mattson at the National Institutes of Health found 12-16 hours of fasting reduced excess body fat.[39] Adnin Zaman, MD. conducted a study finding eating in the evening and at late bed-time is associated with overweight and higher body fat. He found that those who ate within an 11-hour window that extended into the evening hours had weight issues. Therefore, a better weight-loss strategy would be to eat within a 10-hour window starting within 2 hours of waking.[40] The good news is obesity from disrupting the circadian rhythm can be reversed by switching from being an unrestrained eater to one who chooses a reasonable time-restricted meal pattern.[41]

There is currently not enough human research to either support or refute the use of time-restricted fasting as a weight loss method. Research does exist, though, on meal timing involving eating breakfast, which shows a positive relationship between a morning meal and decreased risk of overweight/obesity. A 2013 study, reported in *Obesity*, found that people who ate large breakfasts lost almost 2.5 times the number of pounds and inches off the waist when compared to people who ate large dinners.[42] Most recently, researchers determined there are more calories burned, lower blood sugar and a lower insulin response after a large breakfast when compared to metabolic results after a large dinner of the same calories. Participants of the study also exhibited increased hunger, especially for sweets, throughout the day after a low-calorie breakfast.[43]

Eating breakfast is also a common habit among those who have been successful losing significant weight and have kept it off long term. And yet, it is the meal that is so commonly skipped. Remember that there is more body fat stored from a larger evening meal than from a large breakfast, even when daily calorie intake is the same. Calories eaten later in the day are more easily stored as fat. Some research supportive of a morning meal cites circadian rhythm and higher morning metabolism as to why this is so. Historically, humans developed to eat mostly during the day when we could see our food. Interestingly, hunger is at its lowest point in the morning suppressed by hormones, which seems odd considering that we are mostly fasting during sleep, so one would think we would be ravenous upon waking. So, if forcing ourselves to eat a large breakfast when the desire for food is low and to eat a large dinner that promotes fat storage are both counterproductive, the best strategy is to eat a large lunch or mid-day meal, similar to European cultures.

A small study of young adult women who were breakfast skippers compared food cravings after eating a 350-calorie normal protein (13g) breakfast with a 350-calorie high protein (35g) breakfast and a no-breakfast option for six consecutive days. Both groups of breakfast eaters, but not the breakfast skippers, had reduced post-meal cravings and decreased appetite hormones. The high protein breakfast, though, sustained the greatest lack of interest in food longest, until before lunch.[44] It is useful to experiment on yourself. Keep a journal of your food intake, noting feelings of hunger and fullness throughout the day, and alternating between a normal protein breakfast, a high protein breakfast, and no breakfast at all. Keep in mind, the effects of breakfast impact evening consumption of highly processed, high carbohydrate snack foods, so be aware of all changes in your hunger and craving patterns. Eating breakfast and perhaps not going on another diet, may be just the thing your body needs to shed those extra pounds.

The real challenge people have with diets is that they are hard to follow for very long. Any diet during which you consume fewer calories than you burn will lead to weight loss—if you stick to it. The question here is: Are "fasting" diets easier to stick with? Not so, according to some people who have used them, citing hunger and low energy. Others say it is easy because you know what to expect each day, whether to eat or not. One researcher, Dr. Krista Varady, at the University of Illinois, who has run human trials lasting 8-10 weeks, found that eating a moderately high-fat diet and eating up to 500 calories on fasting days increased adherence. Up to 20% of her subjects found the diet too difficult; the rest adjusted well after a few weeks. According to Dr. Varady, people do not overeat on their feast days to compensate, reasoning that people can only eat 10-15% more than usual.

Is This Diet For You?

The appeal of intermittent fasting may be because it feels like a part-time diet or maybe it is easier to stick with a plan that includes days that are less restrictive. It definitely is not for you if you don't tolerate the extreme hunger, distraction, irritability, lower work performance, headaches, and possible low blood sugar on fast days...although this non-traditional way of dieting can also be easier than a constant calorie restriction.

If you plan to try IF, whether by Time-Restricted, 5:2 or Alternate Day Fast, please keep these valuable tips in mind:

- The quality of the foods consumed on eating days is especially important since those foods are the primary source of vitamins, minerals, antioxidants, protein, and fiber that keep you healthy.

- Eating whatever you want on the non-fast days will lessen your chances of success—you will lose more weight by eating vegetables, fruits, lean protein, and healthy fats on those days.

- Don't skimp on calories. Consuming an insufficient number of calories causes metabolism to slow and sabotages weight-loss efforts.

- As always, be mindful to stay well-hydrated, especially when you are fasting. That means drinking enough water during feasting *and* fasting periods.

- With fasting, as with other food restrictions, there is the temptation to binge as well as to harbor unhealthy fixations on food.

Intermittent fasting is a plan you can ease into so you may be able to adjust your eating habits and maintain the diet longer by starting with a 12/12 eating pattern (eating within a twelve-hour window and abstaining from all food the following twelve hours). This repetitive pattern is the closest to a natural eating pattern, minus the late evening snacking that packs on the pounds. If you are a night owl, simply adjust the twelve-hour eating window to end at 8 or 9 PM. One suggestion that leads to success is to gradually move breakfast time later and later until you get used to going without food from 8 or 9 PM to 9 AM the following day. Slowly adjusting the time of your morning meal will help you determine what works for you.

Fasting can be dangerous for some people and is definitely not suitable for children, pregnant women, or the elderly. Certain medications also make fasting medically unsafe. Individuals with diabetes or hypoglycemia should always avoid going for long periods of time without food. Athletes should be concerned about speed and performance issues.

An American Heart Association statement supporting alternate-day and periodic fasting for short-term weight loss held there is not enough evidence of effectiveness long-term.

The National Institutes of Health, although not endorsing very low-calorie intake, suggests a maximum of 12 weeks using intermittent fasting methods.

Besides being effective for weight loss, research hints that IF may lower blood pressure, inflammation, cholesterol, and triglycerides, as well as increase insulin sensitivity and reduce cancer risk. If this is found to be true through scientific research, intermittent fasting could be a winner. Stay tuned!!

Worth A Try: Although not a long-term solution for everyone, for some people following an intermittent fast for a few days helped them kick-start a healthier eating plan. Overall, the statistics are promising that IF can lead to weight loss and positive health changes. People whose food intake is not driven by hunger may find this diet easy and effective. The change in eating schedule also helps identify mindless eating practices. The flexibility inherent in this method also works well for shift workers or those who travel. It does most certainly increase awareness of world hunger and sympathy for those who do not have consistent access to food.

Pass It By: Fasting is difficult to stick with for most people and for some it is dangerous. Intermittent fasting is never suitable or safe for children, the elderly, or individuals with health issues or on medications. People with diabetes, hypoglycemia, heart disease or hypertension, and pregnant women should always avoid long periods of time without food. The risk of hypoglycemic incidences while fasting is double for people with diabetes who take medication to lower blood sugar.

Supervision by a health professional when planning on using IF is strongly advised.

Detoxification Diets: Cleanses And Juice Fasts

No single specific detoxification diet exists. Although detox methods vary, these diets usually share a common goal, to eliminate the sources of toxins being ingested. This is a technique used to rid the body of foreign substances.

Consider for a moment why people feel the need to detoxify through diet vs. how the body detoxes naturally. The first line of defense against foreign substances is the intestinal wall. The intestinal wall forms the largest immune defense organ that blocks, to some extent, the transfer of damaging compounds into the bloodstream. Furthermore, the liver and kidneys remove toxins and impurities on an ongoing basis without our input.

Everything we absorb into our body, whether through inhalation, ingestion, or through the skin, goes through the liver via the blood. The liver is designed to neutralize toxins and the liver is self-cleaning. There is no evidence that a normal liver fills with toxins, which makes us wonder if the positive effects of detoxing are from the cleanse itself or from the temporary elimination of these substances being poured into the liver.

Or, maybe the cleanse is beneficial by allowing the liver to catch up with the backlog of work it must do. We are most definitely exposed to pollution, chemicals, pesticides, hormones, antibiotics, and irritants, and there are circumstances where detoxifications and cleanses are beneficial, especially when there is a heavy metal buildup as in mercury or arsenic. In these cases, the diets are targeted to ridding the body of a specific substance and are done under medical supervision. On the other hand, the media-driven detox diet does not clinically test hair, blood, or urine to identify the existence of or type of toxins to be eliminated.

How It Works

The typical detox/cleanse diet is about avoiding sugar, alcohol, caffeine, dairy, processed foods, and grains, leaving a diet of only vegetables, fruits, and lean proteins. Mmmm...doesn't sound like most people could stay satisfied or maintain an active lifestyle with such strict limitations long-term. However, a lasting healthy approach to rid the body of toxin overload is to simply avoid or minimize added sugar, alcohol, and caffeine intake, along with eliminating preservatives and food additives, including antibiotics and hormones. Sometimes referred to as "clean eating," this healthy plan does have a huge impact on health and weight loss. Healthy diet options that incorporate "clean eating" principles are DASH (page 89) and the Mediterranean Diet (page 84). Clean eating also eliminates the toxins that have been found to disrupt the endocrine system and natural regulators that act on weight maintenance. Although there is no evidence that fad detox diet plans lead to weight loss, removing toxic substances that impair our natural weight-associated regulators provided by the gut and endocrine system may help you to lose weight by whatever method you choose next.

One popular detox diet involves juicing. A juice fast can last a few days up to a few weeks and often limits eating other food. This results in not only calorie restriction, but nutrient deficiency. This restriction results in weight loss, which is often rapid, and therefore appealing to the impatient dieter. But again, after resuming poor eating habits, the weight returns and often increases. There is further concern for low blood sugar and loss of muscle mass along with electrolyte imbalances.

There are less restrictive detox methods. Follow these suggestions to rid the body of a toxin overload.

- ✓ Choose organic to reduce pesticide and GMO ingestion[45]
- ✓ Eat more plant food for vitamins, minerals, antioxidants, and fiber
- ✓ Eliminate processed foods to reduce consumption of chemicals, preservatives, and food additives
- ✓ Eat fewer animals and, when you do, choose free-range and cage-free animals as well as wild-caught fish to eliminate the hormones and antibiotics conventionally raised animals are treated with
- ✓ Avoid overcooked meat, which produces Advanced Glycation Endpoints (AGEs)
- ✓ Avoid processed food and choose whole foods instead
- ✓ Drink more water to help flush toxins from the body
- ✓ Don't smoke
- ✓ Avoid alcoholic beverages
- ✓ Exercise to improve elimination and to manage abdominal visceral fat, which can damage the liver, the detoxing organ

What The Experts Say

Sometimes a detoxifying plan is needed to purge toxins and impurities from the body, even with a properly working liver. Some people may have an overload of toxins entering the body through the air, food, or skin. With a toxicant-induced loss of tolerance, where the body is overloaded with toxins, the body reacts to much smaller doses of these chemical substances. The increased sensitivity can cause adverse symptoms, which can also impact weight. Brain fog and fatigue can cause an individual to eat more, thinking it is food the body needs to feel better. Sensitivities to foods such as soy, corn, gluten, dairy, etc. can contribute to poor organ function. These issues are best identified and discussed with a nutrition practitioner who will prescribe a personalized protocol specifically designed to address and insure adequate calories and nutrient intake without adverse effects.

There is no evidence that a specific food combination can eliminate toxins from the body. However, this fad has caught on without concern for what is truly safe and healthy. As for weight loss, experts have found no evidence to support the use of detox/cleanse methods for weight management.

In addition, detox plans may not be offering nutritionally sound advice. Some encourage juice two times a day with one meal of whole food, providing too little calories, especially if exercise is involved. Any extreme is fraught with health risks. Some advocates tout detox for more energy and better skin. Was it the juicing or the removal of alcohol, processed carbohydrates and food additives that really did the trick? That being said, juicing may be the kick-start to much needed healthier habits, like increasing fruit and vegetable consumption, shunning fast food and happy hour, and more sleep and yoga. Yet again, it must be pointed out that the effects are short-lived if the deprivation causes a surge in the appetite for forbidden or forgone foods.

Consider eating these whole foods daily to help the body detoxify naturally:
- Alliums: Garlic, leeks, onions, and shallots

- Brassicas: Brussel sprouts, broccoli, cauliflower, cabbage, kale

- Herbs, Spices, Tea: Cilantro, ginger, parsley, oregano, turmeric, mint, rosemary, curry, decaffeinated green tea

- Fruits: Pomegranates, berries, watermelon, grapefruit

- Vegetables: Arugula, beets, red cabbage, mustard greens, artichokes, Swiss chard

Is This Diet For You?

Buyer Beware! Some packaged juice cleanses contain plenty of sugar. And isn't sugar one of the reasons why you are cleansing in the first place? Many prepackaged vegetable juices list pear juice first on the ingredient list, hiding the sugar in a healthy sounding name. When drinking these highly processed juices, along with the fruits and vegetables is a concentrated amount of sugar. (Yes, juice is a processed food). It may be okay in an 8-ounce serving, but many of the drink containers hold 16-24 ounces. Also, when you drink your calories, you are unlikely to compensate for the added calories by consuming less solid food. This means if your drink contains 150 calories a day and you don't eat 150 fewer calories at meals, you can potentially gain 10-15 pounds after a year. That has the same effect on weight, by the way, as drinking a 12-ounce can of soda a day.

Drinking shakes and smoothies may be healthier than juicing in that they usually contain more whole foods processed in a blender and retain more fiber and nutrients. Shakes and smoothies usually contain more protein as well, something that is often inadequate on a juice plan. The increased protein helps preserve lean body mass.

Consider your reasons for detox. Maybe you need a break if you have been eating a lot of processed and packaged foods, have been in contact with too much plastic, which can be toxic, or perhaps are concerned about the amount of antibiotics and hormones in your foods from animal sources. Or maybe a short break from your usual food choices will improve your eating choices and jump-start weight loss. Then I suggest you consider limiting the cleanse to three days for safety. Do not fall prey to marketing hype and use caution. Consuming fewer calories and nutrients means not getting what is required to be considered a balanced meal. There might be weight loss, but with a risk of losing muscle mass, having episodes of low blood sugar, electrolyte imbalances, and a slowed metabolism. These factors commonly lead to weight regain.

Worth A Try: If your meals have been coming more from the drive-thru and your snacks from chip bags and vending machines, you may want to try a detox or cleanse for a few days. It will give you the opportunity to plan how to eat cleaner.

Pass It By: Initial weight loss may be from water weight and quickly regained without further changes away from poor eating habits. Health issues and imbalances also make this diet risky, so first speak with a physician.

Whole30 Diet

The Whole30 diet promotes planning, healthy food choices, and decision-making. The diet is very restrictive, but keep in mind it was created as a short-term diet, a way of understanding how the foods that are eliminated during the 30 days affect cravings, energy, and how you physically feel.

How It Works

Whole30 followers eat three meals a day with no snacking of any kind. Whole30 makes it essential to purchase high quality fresh foods that are limited to meat, seafood, eggs, nuts, seeds, fruits, and vegetables. The goal of this is to help develop an awareness of how foods like sugar, grains, dairy, and alcohol affect weight. Whole30 followers focus on what they are eating and how they are preparing it. These habits are important ones to acquire for successful long-term weight control. The elimination of calories leads to weight loss during the 30 days of the plan, but again, this is not intended as a long-term solution to overweight/obesity and is best followed by another weight loss strategy. Whole30 can easily transition to Mediterranean, DASH, and Volumetrics.

For 30 days, all consumed foods have no added sweetener of any kind, including natural or sugar substitutes. This means none of the usual suspects like sugar, high fructose corn syrup, Splenda, honey, pure maple syrup, sugar alcohols (like sorbitol), as well as the not-so-common sugar sources such as coconut sugar and agave. Carbohydrates are limited to those from fruits and vegetables. Excluded from the plan are all legumes/beans, including soy, lentils, peas and peanuts; all grains, including wheat, rice, corn, oats, barley, quinoa and other gluten-free options; plus all ingredients derived from grains like cornstarch. Yes, folks, that means no cereal, brownies, cookies, pasta, muffins, bread, pizza, and chips. Basically, all baked goods and junk foods must go, even if they are made with Whole30-approved ingredients. You also must remove dairy that comes from all sources, including cows, sheep, and goats. Having no alcohol is cited as one of the hardest rules to follow. Also challenging is the no food-additives rule, hence the need for lots of label reading.

Then comes the second phase. After a full 30 days on the elimination diet, foods are reintroduced slowly to identify those with negative effects on the body, including gas/bloating, headaches, and rashes. Any foods that cause discomfort are eliminated permanently. This phase may take two weeks or longer.

There are no rules for cheating or splurging, they are simply not allowed. The diet recommends that with the slightest slip, including even the smallest amount of restricted foods, you turn the clock back to day one of thirty. This commitment is essential to heal the gut or support the immune system. In this way, Whole30 may make it easier to revamp your diet by providing the appropriate framework in which to do it. Patients often get these same recommendations from their healthcare providers, but sadly, without the tools to help them comply. The Whole30 plan also encourages support from family and friends and the website provides a support network.[46] Considering the 30-50 days the hit takes on your social life, a support system is important for being able to adhere to the plan.

The High Points of Whole30

- Increasing use of foods free of additives, preservatives, and toxins

- Using whole foods that are the least processed and with very few ingredients

- Avoiding packaged convenience foods

- Ridding the dependence on foods that come in boxes and bags

- Preparing meals at home

- Enhancing foods with herbs and spices

- Increasing intake of fruits and vegetables

- Reading food labels

- Promoting a healthy relationship with food

- Emphasizing health and not weight

- Helping to break the sugar habit

- Discovering new and healthy foods

What The Experts Say

Whole30 claims to heal your gut, improve mental health and skin problems, restore metabolic efficiency, and heal the immune system. These claims may very well be true for some with those specific health issues. There is strong research indicating that the removal of some grains, dairy, and sugar can benefit auto-immune diseases, food sensitivities, acne, gut dysfunction (including reflux and irritable bowel syndrome), and inflammatory conditions like arthritis and joint pain. But the diet also claims "total health and food freedom," which is an exaggeration.

A major issue with this plan is that the highly restrictive nature of phase one limits key nutrients vital for optimal health. It is difficult for many people to go such a long time avoiding foods without grain and dairy ingredients. If you have been reading food labels, you are well aware that eliminating grains and legumes also removes those important sources of fiber and B vitamins, and the no-dairy restriction eliminates important sources of calcium and protein. Also to consider, Whole30 encourages the consumption of red meat, pork, coconut oil, and clarified butter, all of which increase saturated fat that is known to compromise heart health.

Is This Diet For You?

Whole30 is an extremely restrictive plan that, as the title indicates, lasts for 30 days. There are a lot of rules specified in the diet and following those rules takes a great deal of planning and preparation in order to get adequate nutrition. It is a big commitment. The diet calls for restarting the 30 days any time you eat *any* of the taboo foods. And yet, the plan is user-friendly, providing extremely specific rules, access to meal-planning guides, and an online community for support.

From a weight loss perspective, any restrictive eating plan with a reduction in calories usually yields results. Yet, when the restriction is not sustainable, the weight returns. Therefore, Whole30 does not necessarily lead to long-term weight reduction. This diet may be a good option if used to jump-start a weight loss effort. Plus, the 30-day restriction can lead to feeling virtuous and empowered resulting from an improved body image, less fatigue (thanks to the absence of high sugar, carb-laden foods), and the acquisition of the tools needed for healthy eating along with promoting a readiness to continue with a less restrictive weight loss plan.

Worth A Try: Whole30 is popular with Crossfit enthusiasts and Paleo diet followers. The unprocessed plant-based whole food approach certainly contributes to improved health. You may not realize sustainable weight loss, but after 30 processed carbohydrate and sugar-free days, I'm betting you will be ready to stick to a more moderate plan and live comfortably without your former indulgences. This one is for you if you can make the commitment, want to clean out the pantry, hope to control sugar and carb cravings, and do well with all-or-none thinking. Whole30 works best for home cooks, planners, and label readers.

Pass It By: Vegetarians will find it difficult to meet the protein needs without beans, legumes, and grains. Individuals with high cholesterol or other heart health risks need to focus more on leaner proteins and healthier fat choices. For those who have a more active social life, who eat out and attend parties, or who travel, following this plan will be extremely challenging. Whole30 is also not budget-friendly and demands the purchase of expensive proteins and produce. If you find meal planning, grocery shopping, and cooking a drag, or if you don't have the time and cannot make the effort this plan requires, you are setting yourself up for frustration and failure—the emotions that are always counterproductive to losing weight.

Mediterranean Diet

The Mediterranean diet is a trend, not a fad, which means it is an established 5000-year-old style of eating that has gained in popularity around the world. Its name comes from the area surrounding the Mediterranean Sea, which includes the countries of Greece, Italy, Spain, Israel, Syria, and Lebanon. The people who live in this part of the globe and follow this diet enjoy some of the best health in the world. Based on years of research, nutrition experts agree that this eating plan leads to weight loss and maintenance. In fact, the Mediterranean diet rated among the top three best overall diets for the last ten years, ranking #1 in 2020, in the *U.S. News and World Report* review of the best diets, for its healthy easy-to-use method of losing weight in both the short- and long-term…and the food is terrific!

How It Works

Mediterranean cuisines use whole grains, vegetables, fruits, lean animal proteins, healthy fats, herbs and spices, nuts and seeds. This eating plan shifts the user away from refined carbohydrates and sugar to whole, unprocessed foods. Mediterranean dishes are a great opportunity to skip the wheat and use barley, buckwheat, and bulgur for whole grains. The high soluble fiber content of these grains means they take longer to digest, thereby suppressing the appetite. Beans, including chickpeas, and legumes, like lentils and peas, are also featured. Healthy fats include olives and olive oil, avocados, almonds, and walnuts. Refined oils and trans fats are discouraged. The message here is healthy fat not low fat. A moderate consumption of alcohol is allowed, especially red wine, with 4 ounces of 100% grape juice recommended as an option for non-drinkers. You will not find large portions of red meat and cheese in this eating style, which also means lower sodium and saturated fat. If you are among those who have already been heeding advice to curb red meat and cheese consumption and up your vegetable game, following a Mediterranean diet may be easier than you think.

Meals of the Mediterranean can be all vegetarian, but they often include fish, calcium-rich yogurt, and lean meats. Dishes that are based on plant-based proteins make meat-free meals possible. The Mediterranean diet is typically at least 30% fat, mostly from olives, olive oil, nuts and seeds, with saturated fat making up no more than 8% of total calorie intake.

Since many cultures contribute to the Med diet, this means a variety of flavors from many different herbs and spices. This is not a boring diet. The Mediterranean plate is full of vegetables, fruits, grains, and pulses (beans and legumes) with just about a third devoted to animal protein, if being included at all. These high nutrient-dense, low-calorie-dense foods are full of fiber and water, increasing satiety with fewer calories.

Transitioning to the Mediterranean style of eating can be done easily and slowly.

- Make meals and snacks from unprocessed foods.

- Replace red meats in meals with fish.

- Substitute ground chicken and turkey for chopped beef.

- In meals, use vegetarian protein options like beans and legumes for healthy meat-free meals.

- Cook more stews and stir fries to increase your intake of vegetables.

- Switch out pretzels and chips snacks with raw veggies and hummus.

- Eat vegetable omelets instead of plain eggs for breakfast.

- Add beans to favorite soup and stew recipes.

- Branch out from ho-hum white rice and make meals interesting with couscous, barley, buckwheat, and faro.

- Use olive oil for cooking and oils derived from nuts and seeds for flavor-filled sauces and dressings.

- Add nuts or seeds to salads or make them your afternoon snack.

- You can use ground nuts to coat fish in place of breadcrumbs.

- Utilize fresh and dried herbs, garlic, onions, and olive oil to add flavor to any dish.

The Mediterranean diet plan includes two precepts not often included in a diet: One is daily physical activity, a way to increase calorie burn and boost metabolism for better weight loss and maintenance. Two is sharing food with family and friends. The Mediterranean diet encourages social support and enjoyment of life whereas many other diets impact lifestyle, isolating the dieter from social situations and challenging eating events.

What The Experts Say

Research from the nineties to the present comparing weight, health risks, and disease development between the typical American and Northern European diet and the Mediterranean diet found the Med way of eating reduced weight, specifically waist circumference (belly fat). The Mediterranean diet was also found to be as effective as a low-carb diet for improvements in blood sugar and cholesterol levels.[47]

The foods in this eating plan consist of those that are classified as minimally processed, full of fiber, anti-inflammatory compounds and healthy fats. All of the foods promote a healthy balance of gut bacteria, and all are supportive of weight loss and good health. This diet also highlights the importance of choosing organic grass-fed free-range animals whenever possible as to avoid ingesting antibiotics, hormones, and toxic chemicals, which have all been found to be endocrine disruptors that contribute to weight gain and poor health, including heart disease.[48] The more closely you follow the Mediterranean diet, the lower your risk of heart disease, as well as high blood pressure, high cholesterol, inflammation, diabetes, midlife memory loss, Alzheimer's Disease, and age-related cognitive decline.[49][50]

In addition, this diet was effective at not only reducing weight but also triglycerides and liver fat, both important factors in reducing metabolic syndrome, diabetes, and fatty liver disease. This is, in part, because long-term adherence to the Mediterranean diet reduces visceral fat, the fat that surrounds the internal organs. This reduction of fat deposits also includes those surrounding the heart, reducing risk of heart disease as well. Another nod to heart health, the high use of olive oil lowers LDL (bad) cholesterol and raises HDL (good) cholesterol.

University College London researchers even found the Mediterranean diet lowered the risk of depression. These health perks could be from consuming fewer processed foods, sugary foods, and meat, therefore reducing inflammation...or because of the higher Omega-3 fatty acids and antioxidant-rich foods' contribution to brain function. And for those of you who, no matter how hard you try, can't get a good night's sleep, going Med reduces insomnia and improves sleep quality and duration. Scientists may not yet know why, but these positive outcomes mean five stars for the Mediterranean diet.[51]

We also know that people who eat a Mediterranean diet lead longer and healthier lives and research confirms it. On a cellular level, when telomeres, the end caps of genetic threads, become shortened, the cells age and break down, allowing diseases to develop, all of which contribute to a shortening of life. Scientists say adherence to the Med diet preserves telomere length and that translates into a longer life with less risk of chronic disease.[52]

Is This Diet For You?

All foods fit in the Mediterranean diet, which is more of an *eating style*, a type of cuisine, than a diet. The weight lost, by eating in this way, is the added perk gained by feeding your body deliciously healthy lean proteins, vegetables, fruits, fats, and high fiber legumes and grains. Think of it as a way to focus on eating sensible portions of great tasting foods without deprivation. In fact, you can even eat pasta. And remember, you won't feel deprived or bored since this style of eating encompasses dishes from many different countries and geographic regions along with their diversity of ingredients and flavors.

The Med style combines well with Alternate Day Intermittent Fasting (see page 66). The Greek religious observance of fasting Wednesdays and Fridays mimics Alternate Day Fasting, which research supports for weight loss, blood sugar control, and longevity. Synching the two eating plans provide a waist-slimming, disease-reducing diet.

Worth A Try: The Mediterranean diet is not restrictive in that it comes down to eating more of what is good for you rather than less of what isn't. Although the foods are mostly unprocessed and not prepackaged, there are healthy foods that come in convenient packaging. Beans and legumes can be purchased already cooked, in cans. Vegetables and fruits can be purchased pre-sliced fresh or frozen. Fish, too, can be purchased fresh or frozen depending on when you plan to cook it. Hunger won't be a problem with the high fiber and healthy fats helping you feel full. Additionally, for those concerned about the environment, the Med diet has a lower water and carbon footprint and promotes sustainable agriculture. This eating style is safe to enjoy by most people.

Pass It By: If you are a die-hard carnivore or your meals are usually something you pick up from the drive-thru, the Mediterranean diet won't appeal to you. If your vegetable and fruit preferences are limited, you may also find it challenging. Where you live or food shop may also limit the availability of certain food items.

Dash Diet

DASH stands for **D**ietary **A**pproach to **S**top **H**ypertension, but don't let the name fool you. DASH is also an effective weight-loss plan. Developed by the National Heart, Lung and Blood Institute, a division of the National Institutes of Health, the DASH diet is especially advantageous to those with high blood pressure; however, *any* adult following this plan can maximize heart health, lower risk of some cancers, and reduce inflammation, which is the root cause of change in the body including aging. In addition, scientific research has generated dramatic results showing that the DASH diet also promotes healthy weight loss. DASH is not a fad, but a well-established eating plan that is gaining momentum. In fact, every year *US News & World Report* ranks the DASH Diet among the top 10 diets for user-friendly weight loss methods. In 2020, it shared the number two spot with the Flexitarian diet (page 94).

How It Works

The DASH diet offers a plan of nutrient-rich, lower calorie-dense foods to support weight loss and weight maintenance. It advocates daily eating of fruits, vegetables, whole grains, nuts, seeds, beans and 6 ounces or less of meat, poultry, or fish a day. Low-fat or fat-free dairy is encouraged to reduce saturated fat intake and promote heart health. Sweets, fatty meats and added fats are limited, not eliminated.

The DASH diet has built-in guidelines for portion control, it encourages variety, and even suggests the occasional sweet treat. The recommended number of servings for each food group will vary based on calorie requirements.

What To Eat On DASH [53]

Food Group	Number of Servings	Examples of 1 Serving
Grains	6-8 servings/day	1 slice bread, 1 oz cereal, ½ cup brown rice
Vegetables	4-5 servings/day	1 cup leafy vegetables, ½ cup cooked broccoli
Fruit	4 servings/day	1 whole fruit, ½ cup frozen or canned fruit, ½ cup juice
Low-fat or fat-free milk products	2-3 servings/day	1 cup milk, 8 oz yogurt, 1½ oz cheese
Lean meats, poultry, and fish	2 or less servings/day	3 oz cooked chicken/fish/meat, 1 egg
Legumes, beans, nuts, and seeds	4-5 servings/week	½ cup lentils, ¼ cup nuts, 2 tbsp nut butter
Fats, oils	2-3 servings/day	1 tsp oil, 1 tbsp salad dressing
Sweets and added sugars	5 or less servings/week	1 tbsp jelly, 1 tbsp sugar, 1 small cookie

What The Experts Say

The weight loss is a result of eating plant-based and low-fat foods that have a lower calorie density (See Volumetrics Diet pg. 54). With a plate full of vegetables and fruits, you wind up eating fewer calories. So, if you're wondering why the DASH diet hasn't caught on, it may be because it was designed and promoted to prevent disease and optimize health. With a little rebranding and a celebrity endorsement, this diet could really take off. If you are interested in following this plan, check out the DASH app to make it easy.

The challenge for people used to a lifestyle of fast food is that following the DASH diet means replacing a trip to the fast food drive-through with a trip to the market for groceries that need to be prepared or assembled at home. However, before you give up on this diet, consider today's wide array of healthy convenience items found in your supermarket or grocery store. Vegetables, frozen or fresh, already pre-sliced/chopped, found in the produce aisle may just become your new fast food. Frozen pre-cooked shrimp and canned fish are an easy way to replace meats with healthier fish and seafood. Canned beans and legumes need no cooking time but should be rinsed before use to remove added salt.

Another obstacle to popularizing the DASH diet might be the cost. One study found that food costs were 18% higher. If cost is a concern, consider buying fruits and vegetables in season and in bulk to save some money. Look for "ugly" produce in your market. Those misshapen runts are just as tasty and nutritious as their beautifully developed sibs and are sold at a significantly lower price.

Also, adherence to DASH is more environmentally friendly because it reduces greenhouse gas production, ultimately reducing the cost of food on our planet.

One thing to be aware of is that if you are not used to eating plant fruits, vegetables, and whole grains, you will need to add these foods slowly and increase the amount you eat very gradually. A sudden increase in plant foods can cause temporary bloating and diarrhea until the body becomes accustomed to processing the increased fiber. But it is temporary and better for you in the long run. The following are ways to make gradual changes and inclusions to introduce vegetables and fruits into your diet.

The Best Ways To DASH

- Eat a serving of fruit instead of cookies, or cake, or candy, when you crave something sweet

- Snack on raw veggies dipped in low-fat dressing or hummus instead of chips and high-calorie dips when you want a crunchy snack

- Snack on ¼ cup dried fruit and nut mix and skip the typical snack foods with their processed carbs and added sugars

- Snack on popcorn, just watch the sodium content

- Make vegetables half of your lunch and dinner meals; soups and stews are an easy way to do this

- Substitute ground white-meat turkey for ground beef in burgers, meat loaf, tacos, and chilis

- Choose low-fat or fat-free condiments such as mustard or hummus on your sandwich instead of mayo or dressing

- Halve the amount of cooking oils and fats

- Add fruit (fresh or frozen) to plain yogurt to reduce the sugar content

- Switch from soda (even diet soda) to water or flavored seltzer

- Limit all foods with added sugar, including baked goods, candy, ice cream, fruit-flavored yogurts, sherbets, cereal, and breakfast/snack bars

- Use fresh or frozen instead of canned vegetables; if using canned products, make sure they are the no-salt-added or reduced-sodium variety (read the label)

- Choosing frozen fruits and vegetables may be more cost effective than fresh

- Eat whole grain breads, whole grain cereals, wild rice, quinoa, barley, buckwheat, and other alternate grains

- Include a lean protein-rich food at all meals

- Snacks should include a protein-rich food along with a serving of fruit or vegetable, i.e. hard-boiled egg, cheese, milk/yogurt, nuts

For more ideas on how to use the DASH eating plan, visit the National Institutes of Health website and search keywords DASH diet.[54]

Is This Diet For You?

The DASH diet removes the restrictions and "all or none" thinking that trips up many dieters. The health benefits of the DASH diet are profound, with positive results seen even without 100 percent adherence. This is helpful in breaking the mentality of "being on a diet" and following strict rules, then "going off" and undoing past efforts. This is a refreshing and encouraging alternative that allows you to do your best and not be concerned about getting it all perfect while still seeing results and establishing healthier food behaviors necessary for long-term success. It truly is more like an easy paced stroll then a dash to the finish line.

For those who prefer full-fat cheese and yogurt and perhaps a bit more meat, the good news is that a recent study, reported in the *American Journal of Clinical Nutrition*, found a reduction in disease risk despite increased fat intake above DASH levels while adhering to the other DASH recommendations. Be aware, though, that higher fat consumption also means more calories and may impact weight loss.

Worth A Try: DASH is a "slam-dunk" if you want to lose weight, clean up your diet, improve blood pressure, cholesterol, and heart health. The rules are easy to follow and include all types of food, making this plan useful in realizing a permanent change in your food habits and your weight.

Pass It By: If you have been plagued by intestinal issues, bloating, gas, or diarrhea, consult a physician before adding high fiber foods to your diet. They could make symptoms worse.

Flexitarian Diet

Developed by Dawn Jackson Blatner in 2009, the Flexitarian diet, is taking the diet community by storm. Its draw is its lack of rules, a refreshing change from diets like Atkins and Whole30 with their food restrictions. In fact, the Flexitarian diet is so healthy and easy to use that it was a tie for second place in *US News and World Report* Best Diets 2020. The Flexitarian style of eating encourages a plant-based diet without eliminating meat completely. Weight loss results from cutting calories by eating more vegetables and fruits. Think of it as Vegetarian lite. Blatner coined the phrase based on flexible vegetarians, those who go meatless most of the time. Vegetarians eliminate most foods derived from animals, but some may include dairy and eggs. Vegans completely avoid eating all animal-based foods.

How It Works

The premise is that all foods can be eaten but the goal is to replace animal foods with plant-based options 2-5 days per week. All meals are comprised of vegetables, fruits, grains, bean, legumes, nuts, and seeds. Flexitarians also rely on tofu and other soy-based proteins along with beans and lentils to meet their protein needs. Followers are encouraged to avoid processed foods in favor of whole or minimally processed plant-based foods, typically lower in calories. Additionally, the Flexitarian diet limits added sugars and sweet snacks.

A major perk of this method is the ease of the transitioning toward vegetarian. Beginners usually start with two meatless days per week or even one day at a time, even one meal at a time. Those that embrace the lifestyle can eat vegetarian five or more days per week. Because of the flexibility, this weight loss method is compatible with health-related dietary restrictions such as gluten-free or allergens, as well as individual food preferences as long as they include vegetables and fruits. There is also no calorie limit, so weight loss is dependent on being self-aware of portion sizes.

What The Experts Say

Evident in most research on effective weight loss is the promotion of increasing intake of vegetables, fruits, whole grains, and pulses. The eating of plant-based diets crowds out animal-derived foods and packaged meals and snacks and replaces them with healthier lower calorie options. Weight loss on the Flexitarian diet is similar to weight loss after having switched to a vegan or vegetarian diet, all examples of reducing or eliminating animal-derived foods.[55] Keep in mind that without going totally vegetarian, weight loss results will vary and are not expected to equal those of vegans or vegetarians. However, going Flexitarian is an easy way to make the change to a more plant-based diet. The lack of rules is not always a benefit. Some need a more structured plan with help in limiting size of food portions. The Flexitarian eating plan is also a good choice for weight maintenance or when a pause is needed between restrictive diet programs.

Going Vegetarian or Flexitarian can even improve more than your waistline. Researchers have found that the five places on the globe where inhabitants live the longest and healthiest lives are all where a plant-based diet is the primary way of eating. Called Blue Zones, the only one in the U.S. is Loma Linda, CA, where people live an average 10 years longer than other Americans. This area includes vegans, vegetarians, and also lacto-ovo vegetarians (who eat dairy and eggs), and pescatarians (who eat fish/seafood). A Flexitarian diet follower may well enjoy not only more years in life and but also more life in those years.

Is This Diet For You?

The unlimited variety of plant foods guarantees you will never get bored on this eating plan. When you also add the myriad of cooking methods and flavorings, the Flexitarian style is easily tailored to most food preferences thereby increasing the likelihood of sticking with it. Those with limited experience cooking or eating vegetarian or who need new recipe ideas can find support online. A knowledge of plant-based proteins and meat alternatives is also important for optimal nutrition status. Aside from naturally occurring plant proteins, newer options on supermarket shelves, such as Beyond Meat and Gardein, provide protein-rich meat alternatives derived from pea and soy. This flexible plan is also attractive if you travel or frequently eat out.

Worth A Try: Even though buying more produce will add to your food bill, it will be offset by the money you will save on meat. Trying Flexitarian means you are open to experimenting with soy and pea protein sources, and there is a bounty of recipes to be found in Blatner's books along with online resources.[56] [57]

Pass It By: If you are a carnivore or detest vegetables, this plan is not for you. Prepared foods are discouraged so you need to know your way around the kitchen.

Weight Watchers (myWW, WW Freestyle)

At first, I questioned whether to include this ubiquitous weight loss plan as a diet strategy. It is so well known and popular. I also wondered if I could provide a comprehensive explanation based on the fact that there is so little written and researched on the subject. It seems so odd that this method has been used successfully by so many but studied by so few. Then, I happened to be out with some friends for lunch when one of them shared that she was on Weight Watchers and proceeded to order the same grilled chicken with vegetables salad and dressing as I did but without the sweet potatoes and proclaiming her lunch choices as all free foods and no points that sparked my interest as to whether or not Weight Watchers users really were successful at long-term weight loss.

How It Works

The Weight Watchers plan gives users a way to chart calories while advocating healthy food choices and a healthy lifestyle. Support is provided with guidance on preparing healthy meals, and coaching by email or text, or at in-person meetings. Surveys showed that participants lost more weight attending meetings than other support options. Weight Watchers has no forbidden foods and the absence of restricted foods makes it a healthy plan. There are no requirements to purchase their trademark foods or meals, but supermarket shelves are full of Weight Watchers manufactured and endorsed foods. Their Freestyle plan works by assigning Smartpoints to foods, based on their nutrient profile, while also providing the user with a list of "free foods," those deemed to not count toward their prescribed daily point allotment. There are no calories to count, but portion control is imperative if you want to lose weight. Healthier foods are given the lowest points. Being able to assign points to foods with the option to rollover leftover points to another day is a great way to incorporate individual food and lifestyle choices, allow for social eating, and increase adherence to the assigned daily point goals.

What The Experts Say

Free foods encourage eating vegetables and fruits, which increases the intake of fiber to promote fullness, gut health, and the necessary vitamins and minerals for overall health. Most of the foods on the free foods list are vegetables and fruit. I did find it perplexing to also find peas, beans, and lentils on this free list, given that these foods add considerable calories and carbohydrates, albeit healthy ones—if not eaten in carefully controlled portions. Lean proteins also appear on the free list, including chicken breast, turkey, fish, and eggs. A meal of 4 ounces of chicken and 1 cup of lentils would already contain a substantial 300 calories even before adding cooking fats, vegetables, and flavors. One more nod to the importance of portion control for weight loss, regardless of quality of the ingredients.

Weight Watchers also gives the user credit for physical activity, encouraging a healthier lifestyle and increasing the likelihood of maintaining lost weight. The simplicity of this program makes it easy to follow and to stick with.

Results of a study of people 1-5 years after losing weight on Weight Watchers found that, overall, there was a regain of weight between 31.5% and 76.5%. At 5 years, less than 20% were near their goal weight, but 70% were still below their initial weight. Weight Watchers could be a good option for some people.[58] A study that ran from 2000-2002 comparing Ornish, Atkins, Zone, and Weight Watchers found little difference in the amount of weight lost in all the methods with amount of weight lost dependent more on diet adherence than the method used. Again, a diet is only successful if you stick to it.[59]

A 2005 review of major commercial weight loss programs in the U.S. found Weight Watchers ahead of the pack with the largest reported weight loss of 3.2% of initial weight after two years. For the average American woman, 168 pounds, that means losing a little over 5 pounds after two years of dieting. For an average 196-pound American male, that means a total of 6 pounds. When considering Weight Watchers, the question you need to ask yourself is how adherent will you be to this plan and will losing 5-6 pounds make you feel successful.[60]

Is This Diet For You?

The spokesperson for a recent television commercial for the Weight Watchers Freestyle program said, "I lost 82 pounds and I can eat whatever I want." Don't be misled by claims like this. If it sounds too good to be true, it usually is.

Worth A Try: The Weight Watchers plan is easy to use with both online and in person support options. The pervasiveness of the diet plan in the U.S. makes it easy to follow given the number of products that include Weight Watchers information on the label. Like other healthier diet plans, Weight Watchers advocates increased vegetable, fruit, and lean protein intake and not the elimination of any food or food group.

Pass It By: Successful weight loss on Weight Watchers means that attention must be paid to food quality and portion sizes. For those needing a plan with more structure, the free food concept could be a minefield. For those on a budget, Weight Watchers is a pricey option.

Nutrisystem And Jenny Craig

How It Works

Both Nutrisystem and Jenny Craig offer prepackaged meals and snacks making menu planning easy along with the benefit of structure and convenience.

Nutrisystem delivers their food products and provides meal plans and grocery lists for five days. According to the company's research team, Nutrisystem products provide for 60% of daily calories, expecting the additional 40% to come from food obtained from grocery shopping or restaurant meals. They also offer support through a call center as well as a blog and app for food and exercise tracking.

Jenny Craig is prepackaged delivered meals and snacks targeting people who want to lose 16 pounds or less. This personalized plan, developed by dietitians and nutritionists, is designed to result in a steady weight loss of one to two pounds per week. An app is available to track food intake and exercise. The company recently added a Rapid Results Program that uses the body's circadian rhythm to burn more calories. Individual counseling is available by telephone with trained consultants.

What The Experts Say

Although Nutrisystem claims a 7.5% loss from starting weight after six months, no long-term independent studies exist to prove the weight loss is permanent.

There are no published studies supporting any of the claims made by Jenny Craig.

Is This Diet For You?

While you may be able to drop some weight quickly, without a follow-up plan in place, it is likely you will regain the weight. Furthermore, relying on the purchased, proportioned, calorie-controlled foods teaches you nothing about eating appropriately to maintain the weight loss once you are no longer participating in the program. Cost is a factor you need to take into consideration when deciding to use these plans. Their ready to eat foods may run $14-$20 per day in addition to enrollment and maintenance fees.

Meal Replacements

Liquid meal replacements have been a dieting option for the past 50 years. Nutrition bars were introduced in 1986 with the Power Bar marketed to athletes. Combined, meal replacements represent a $4.7

billion share of the diet industry. The term "meal replacement" refers to any prepackaged product in the form of a bar or beverage that is consumed in place of a meal. The meal-replacement industry has changed significantly from past product formulation and selection resulting in increased variety. Choices today include high-protein, low-carb, and organic offering many new flavors. Products vary in calorie content, ranging from 200-400 calories per serving. If you're not careful these meal replacements can be nothing more than glorified liquid candy or candy bars containing high amounts of sugar, sometimes 20 grams.

Liquid meal replacements are often processed carbohydrates and fat, and a meal replacement in liquid form can be upwards of 50% of total daily calories appropriate for weight loss. Meal replacements, in general, provide adequate protein, often 10-20g per serving. Medifast and Slimfast are among the most well-known brands but Orgain, Shakeology, Herbalife and Isagenix have gained in popularity.

How It Works

These are marketed as replacements for all or a part of a meal. Successful weight loss occurs most often when the product is used as a total meal. It is popular to use these meal replacements for one or two meals a day and making the balance of meals with whole foods. Some users rely on meal replacement products as a health-conscious convenient food that prevents overeating.

What The Experts Say

Studies supporting the use of meal replacements for weight loss usually come from the manufacturers of these products who have a stake in their success.[61] One independent clinical trial showed that the use of a nutritionally sound liquid meal replacement resulted in greater weight loss than a food-based diet. A study of Optifast published in the journal *Obesity* found two-thirds of participants were able to sustain weight loss at 52 weeks.[52] Another recent study found that participants using meal replacements for a severe calorie restriction over 4 months, followed by 8 months of moderate calorie restriction, lost *twice* as much weight and fat in a year compared with those using a food-based moderate calorie-restricted diet for 12 months.[63] Severe calorie-restricted diets did not impose a greater threat to muscle mass when compared to moderate calorie-restricted plans. Severe calorie restriction, however, does increase risk of bone loss and, therefore, needs to be evaluated and potentially avoided by postmenopausal women, especially those diagnosed with osteopenia or osteoporosis.

Review of multiple studies have led experts to conclude that meal replacements are an easy-to-use, well tolerated, and effective tool for weight loss. In addition, the research suggests that meal replacement beverages do cause a person to feel fuller while keeping calories low. Another advantage to using liquid meal replacements is they are often fortified with vitamins, minerals, and other nutrients that are lacking in other methods relying on limited food intake. These findings offer support of this method for successful long-term weight management.

Is This Diet For You?

If you find pre-portioned meal replacements helpful, this takes the work out of creating your own meals that meet specific calorie and nutrient specifications. The disadvantage is boredom from the repetitive taste and texture. However, research also suggests that this decreased pleasure may actually lead to reduced appetite and calorie intake. The one clear negative to liquid meal replacements is the real possibility of nutrient deficiencies, most notably fiber, which can lead to constipation. One way to assure adequate fiber intake is to add fruits and vegetables to the plated meals required in this plan. Some of these products contain an inadequate supply of unprocessed carbohydrates and too much sugar, which may result in low energy and food cravings.

Look for products that contain at least 20g protein and low in added sugar. Avoid the products that claim to boost energy as they usually contain caffeine or other stimulants.

Also, it's important to remember that this method relies on low food intake during the day that can lead to night eating, adding to the total daily calories and hindering weight loss. A major disadvantage to this type of weight-loss plan is the lack of education about realistic portion sizes and the ability to recognize the signs of hunger and fullness, making the transition back to a whole food diet problematic for sustaining any weight loss. Do not be fooled by claims on the labels. These products do not contain all the nutrients of real food. The vitamins and minerals may be synthetic and if you read the ingredient list you will probably find lots of chemicals.

The biggest advantage is convenience, truly little or no preparation required, and many come in a grab-and-go container.

Worth A Try: If this method appeals to you, I suggest trying it out for 4-6 weeks while you choose the method you will use next. Consult with your physician about potential health risks.

Pass It By: Many meal replacements contain sugar alcohols, which cause bloating and diarrhea in intolerant individuals. Some even contain artificial sweeteners that are known to negatively affect weight. The lack of fiber can cause constipation. Even the synthetic fiber in nutrition bars can cause digestive problems. Following a severe calorie restriction can have long-term consequences for bone health. Another deterrent is that most meal replacement programs hit the wallet pretty hard.

Chapter 4:
New And Noteworthy Trending Diets

The following are diets that are trending and making headlines. It seems like every week a new diet or a new study is in the news, some credible, some incredible (and not in a good way). What follows are the new and noteworthy ideas and research that show promise in winning the war against the battle of the bulge. To help you keep these in perspective, I've attempted to lay out the facts and methods for each one, along with the supporting research whenever possible. Keep in mind that, in many cases, these dietary practices are too new to be backed by sufficient research as to their effectiveness, safety, and long-term results. In light of this absence of expert opinions, it's difficult to make recommendations on every one of them at this time.

CICO (Calories In, Calories Out)

This new weight-loss fad is basically good old calorie counting. Even though the concept is not new, it is tremendously popular on the internet as it promises that you can eat whatever you want and lose weight. The premise is that it doesn't matter if you are consuming soda and chips or vegetables and yogurt as long as you limit daily calories.

How It Works

CICO follows the principle that weight loss occurs when more calories are burned than consumed. Expectations are that all that is needed is the calorie deficit which, in truth, is the basis of most diet plans as science has proven that eating fewer calories than expended results in weight loss. The first step in using CICO is to figure out how many calories you need per day and then subtract 500 calories to give you the number of calories you need to eat every day to lose weight. Those who support it say that it is adherence to the calorie limit that leads to weight loss.

To accurately determine daily calorie goal, you first need to establish how many calories you burn. Devices, trackers, and apps are the most convenient way to do this but may be problematic since not all are accurate. Plus, you can inadvertently log fewer calories than you in fact eat and record more calorie burning exercise than performed. The best option is to use more than one method of record keeping and use an average to increase reliability.

Is This Diet For You?

Because CICO is based on the premise that only calories matter, the danger is that you may continue to make unhealthy food decisions which won't bode well in the long run. Weight regain after this type of dieting is common since improved eating habits were never established. Also, focusing only on quantity without regard for quality guarantees a set-up for nutrient deficiencies. These deficiencies don't seem important in the moment, but the detrimental impact they have on sustainable weight loss and even long-term health is very real. Diet plans with long-term success are the ones that encourage healthy choices of protein to preserve muscle mass (aka lean body mass), because muscle burns the most calories and revs metabolism (the rate at which calories are burned). Losing muscle mass slows weight loss or weight is regained. However, preserving metabolism during weight loss keeps the weight off.

Worth A Try: CICO is a good short-term method for losing a few pounds before an upcoming event or to knock off the extra holiday pounds, but probably will not lead to appreciable long-term sustainable weight loss.

Carb Cycling

Carb Cycling is tailored to athletes and high-intensity exercisers as a way to combine low-carb dieting with carb-loading for energy. This diet is based on alternating between periods of low carbohydrate intake with higher carbohydrate intake. If you find the ketogenic diet explanation confusing, this dieting concept is not for you.

How It Works

There is no specific definition of carb cycling because it is a way to personalize and adjust your own carbohydrate intake based on your specific needs during part of a week, month, or training season. Carb cycling is becoming popular among dieters who have trouble sustaining a low-carb diet and it's easy to see why. Low carbohydrate days are less challenging and easier to maintain when you have a higher carbohydrate period to look forward to. Carb cycling also relieves some of the side effects of severe carbohydrate restriction including constipation, headache, and brain fog. Carb cycling also allows for eating higher carbs on weekends and lower carbs on Monday through Friday or alternating high carb with low carb days throughout the week. In fact, Carb Cycling is especially helpful to those on the Ketogenic diet who exercise regularly and need more carbohydrates for fuel on training days. Choosing to increase carbohydrate intake before and after intense workouts yields better results. Simply put, carbohydrates (hopefully those that are minimally processed and full of fiber) eaten on training days replace some of the fat in the Keto meals. In order to continue in ketosis, this one day of eating carbs must be followed by three or more consecutive low carb days.

What The Experts Say

There is currently no research supporting carb cycling as a viable weight loss method. There is also no evidence of its safety. Because of the negative health consequences inherent in both high and low carb diets, experts recommend a moderate carbohydrate intake.

Is This Diet For You?

It is tricky to keep daily track of carb, fat, and protein needs and it takes a lot of planning.

Worth A Try: If you are using the ketogenic diet and are having issues with energy or performance during exercise, carb cycling may be a solution. Carb cycling may be a useful weight loss approach for frequent travelers who find dieting a challenge when away from home.

Pass It By: Low carb diets decrease energy levels and make it difficult to exercise, and therefore, burn enough calories. The possible side effects of carb cycling are headaches, difficulty concentrating, fatigue, poor fluid balance, and nutrient deficiencies. To be successful and safe, please consult a registered dietitian nutritionist.

Souping

Souping is on its way to replace juicing as the cleanse and jump-start diet of choice and this makes me positively thrilled. Souping is based on the same idea as juicing—replacing traditional meals with liquid-based foods.

How It Works

This hot trend is not a new idea considering the longevity of Volumetrics. Soup, whether eaten for every meal for several days or for one meal a day over time, works by reducing calorie density while still providing the texture and consistency that is so satisfying, helping you eat fewer calories than a meal of solid food. The thicker the soup, like split pea and butternut squash, the better. Another perk of souping is that it takes longer to eat than drinking juices and smoothies. Eating slower is proven to increase satiety and reduce calorie intake.

What The Experts Say

A 2005 study in *Obesity Research* found that people who ate the same number of calories from soup as their counterparts did from chips and pretzels lost 50% more weight.[64] Souping, unlike juicing, does not eliminate or destroy nutrients in the food through processing. Soup also provides a great vehicle for consuming a variety of health boosting, whole foods while restricting calorie intake. Juices contain high amounts of sugar whereas soups, especially those containing vegetables, beans, and lentils, provide complex carbohydrates along with fiber, protein, herbs and spices for a more nutrient-packed, low sugar cleanse or diet alternative.

Is This Diet For You?

The availability of high-quality soup choices from restaurants, delis, and delivery services is growing. However, a word of caution to consider. Soup is notoriously high in sodium, which can impact blood pressure and/or the number on the scale due to water retention. Also be aware that eating soups that are low in calories as meal replacements may mean not getting enough calories. On the flip side, do avoid cream-based soups, which are high in fat, as they add calories and affect weight loss. Buying soups from small storefront restaurants means not having nutrition facts for their menu items. Instead, try delivery services such as www.splendidspoon.com that has an array of soup choices with 4-5 grams fiber, 5-7 grams protein and less than 500 mg sodium each. www.ginacucina.com also offers several healthy soup options. Check the websites.[65][66] Bon Appetit!

Military Diet (AKA 3-Day Diet)

The Military Diet has no connection to any branch of military service and, as far as I can determine, was not developed by any type of credentialed health professional. The Military Diet is a form of intermittent fasting, diet for 3 days and take 4 days off. The diet claims their meal menus, totaling 1100-1400 calories per day, are food combinations that provide energy, control sugar cravings, burn fat, and increase metabolism, yet there is no scientific proof validating these claims. These menus are typical of those used in diets 50 years ago: grapefruit, cottage cheese, saltine crackers, hard boiled eggs, toast, and plain tuna. Water and herbal teas are encouraged, artificial sweeteners are discouraged. Suggested calorie intake on the 4 days off, is 1500/day. The website warns that the user <u>will</u> experience hunger. The diet also brags about being cheap, but of course, you aren't buying much food if you are starving.

What The Experts Say

Calorie restriction causes fatigue, not increased energy, as the Military Diet website claims. Although exercise is important to maintain weight and health, it is ill-advised to do anything strenuous while on this diet which recommends eating only three very regimented meals each day, and no snacks. Calorie intake is the same for everyone at any weight. It does not teach healthy eating habits or the portion control necessary for long-term weight loss. What's more is that the cycle of starvation days can slow metabolism making weight loss more difficult on any future diet plan you choose to follow.

Is This Diet For You?

Worth A Try: Best to keep expectations low. You will lose weight because of the calorie restriction. but you won't keep it off. If your intent is to drop a few for a wedding next weekend, go for it. You will lose water not fat. There is little harm you can do in 3 days, but be prepared for a big disappointment come Monday morning weigh-in. Foods are easy to find, but you won't be eating out on this diet. The minimal meal prep may be a bonus for some.

Pass It By: The Military Diet is not for permanent weight loss. The limited variety of allowed foods will cramp the lifestyle that includes social eating and travel.

Intuitive Eating

Intuitive eating, first described in 1995 by registered dietitians Evelyn Tribole and Elyse Resch, is gaining in popularity at a rapid pace. Intuitive eating, a type of mindful eating, is having an awareness of what you are eating, how much you are eating, and why you are eating. Intuitive eating recognizes that eating is not just a human instinct, but also involves thoughts and feelings as well. It eliminates the feeling that there is a right way and a wrong way to eat. Intuitive eaters do not overeat. Intuitive eaters make healthy, nutritious food choices. That means that even food that is perceived to be unhealthy, when portion controlled, has less of an impact on weight and wellness. Intuitive eaters naturally take in fewer calories without diet instruction and restriction.

What The Experts Say

It is a research proven method to heal negative relationships with food and disrespect for the body. To date, there are over 900 Certified Intuitive Eating Counselors worldwide trained in Intuitive Eating methodology to assist you. Alternatively, you can learn more by reading *Intuitive Eating* by Evelyn Tribole, MS, RDN, CEDRD-S and Elyse Resch MS, RDN, CEDRD-S, FIAEDP, FADA, FAND.[67]

Is this Diet For You?

Yes!

Optavia

Optavia is the latest meal replacement program from the Medifast line. Having the same nutrient profile as the original Medifast products, on the surface, the products seem to be a rebranding marketing ploy. The one difference is that the Optavia plan offers coaching but, important to note, those coaches are paid based on how many meal replacement products they sell to customers on the weight-loss plan. These meal replacement products are called "fuelings." Five servings per day of these fuelings are to be eaten every day and they include high protein soups, bars, biscuits, and puddings, and one meal you need to prepare on your own that includes lean protein, healthy fat, and three servings of vegetables. Daily calorie intake is between 800 to 1000 calories and is considered extremely low, too low in fact to be followed without medical supervision. Optavia also has alternative plans that include more calories that are specifically geared for teens, nursing moms, seniors, and people with health issues. Company-reported weight loss averages one pound per week.

What The Experts Say

US News and World Report ranked Optavia #12 in their category Best Weight-Loss Plans. The high protein content is adequate for preserving muscle mass that is otherwise lost on such a highly restrictive plan. Studies conducted or sponsored by Medifast showed almost half the subjects lost at least 5% of their baseline body weight, and 28% lost a minimum of 10% of their initial weight after 16 weeks on either Optavia or Medifast, the more successful being the dieters who completed more coaching sessions.[68]

Worth a try: This meal replacement program has led to successful weight loss, but you probably won't keep it off.

Pass it by: Be wary of companies and their representatives that profit solely from selling you their products and the coaching you need to stay on this plan. Be prepared for a substantial weight loss from your wallet. A three-week supply of Optavia products costs $350-$425.

Home-Prepared Meals

There is a lower incidence of obesity, 26% to be exact, among people who eat mostly home-prepared meals and don't eat them in front of the TV compared to those who eat out or order take-out, which adds about 200 calories per day. There are many reasons for this discrepancy beginning with the fact that restaurant portions tend to be larger and contain added sugar and fat. Eating out also encourages consumption of sugar-sweetened beverages, dressings and sauces that are easily ordered. Studies have shown these same results whether eating fast food or dining in a fine dining restaurant. The U.S. Centers for Disease Control found that more than 36% of adults eat at least one high-calorie fast food meal every day.

And it is not just fast food meals contributing to obesity. Restaurant food simply contains more calories. This is illustrated in a study published in 2015 that cited an average of 1205 calories per meal in non-chain restaurants. The highest calorie meals hailed from American, Italian, and Chinese restaurants with an average of 1495 calories per meal. You are much better off with a simple home-prepared meal that takes no longer to prepare than ordering and waiting for a take-out delivery.

This makes it clear that the more you eat out or order take-out the easier it is to gain weight and that replacing some or most meals with those prepared at home can reduce or reverse weight gain. Of course, I'm not implying that you should reach for the box of pasta and a jar of sauce for dinner, or cereal and muffins for breakfast. Instead, stock up on convenience foods such as pre-chopped and frozen vegetables, quick cooking whole grains, and canned beans.

Meal Kits

This convenient way of preparing meals at home is available through on-line grocery shopping and meal kit delivery services. There are over one hundred companies nationwide that provide recipes, planning tools, or meal kits to make cooking at home easier and simpler than ever before. Today's meal kits include the pre-measured ingredients and the recipe to easily prepare and get the meal on the table with a minimum of fuss and time. Pre-measured, pre-cut, and prewashed ingredients make home cooked meals easy for anyone seeking convenience, including those lacking cooking skills. Even supermarkets, including Kroger's, Shoprite, and Giant Foods, now have meal kits available to capture a share of the market from meal delivery subscription programs, often at a lower price. Because supermarkets don't require you to pay for a subscription, it is easier to use the service as needed instead of making a commitment ahead of time. Meal kits from supermarkets trend highest among young single men and families with children.

Simple, delicious, and healthy meals are not only quickly prepared, you can choose your meals to match special dietary needs, kitchen skills, and taste preferences. Almost as easy as ordering in! However, even if you feel you don't have time for a grocery run, you lack the skills and confidence to prepare meals, or are just bored with your current options, there are companies providing solutions for every challenge. And this is a good thing because meal delivery kits also encourage skipping restaurants and take-out in favor of healthier and more cost-effective meals. Delivery meal kit services like Blue Apron, Plated, and Hello Fresh raked in about $4 billion in U.S. sales in 2020, showing a strong and growing trend. Meal kits can seem expensive, but when you consider the money saved in food waste, gas to and from the market or restaurant, and throwing away spoiled food or leftovers, meal kits may be the more economical option after all.

Gain some kitchen confidence by using market delivery services like Fresh Direct, Amazon Fresh, Peapod, or any curb-side grocery pick-up, and use the meal-kit recipes and kitchen skills you acquired in preparing well balanced, tasty meals on your own.

On-Line Grocery Shopping

Food shopping online is also an option if you are pressed for time. But beware, it can be either a marvel or a dieting minefield. Before you plug your grocery list into your computer keep the following in mind:

- It will cut down on unhealthy impulse purchases.

- You can be specific about the type and brand of items you want, even the produce.

- Break down large packages into smaller ones to improve portion control including cereal and other processed foods purchased in bulk.

- Plan meals a week (or two) ahead making it easy to have the food on hand you need for both meal prep and grab-and-go options.

Menu Planning

Watch a few cooking shows or on-line videos. Cooking isn't difficult and can be very rewarding to both your ego and your waistline. There are several sites to help you with meal planning using your new or improved kitchen skills. Here's how they work:

- Some sites only provide recipes, others allow you to also save your own recipes

- Most of these sites can generate a shopping list for ingredients

- There are subscription services that email weekly dinner menus that link to grocery shopping online to help you plan ahead

- The online recipes most often contain nutrition facts

- You can choose online recipes that cater to dietary needs, including gluten-free, dairy-free, organic

Good places to start your search
https://elanaspantry.com/gathered-table/
www.hellofresh.com
www.mealboard.com
www.skinnytaste.com

Many supermarket chains also offer recipes and linked shopping lists, so check out the website of your local supermarket. As I write this, I find it curious that the rapid rate of technological advancement has not yet progressed to the kitchen. I dream of smart refrigerators and pantries that are able to keep track of stock and generate shopping lists and also devise meal options based on their contents. Techies out there, are you listening?

Food Journals, Apps, and Gadgets

Food Journals

Self-monitoring is an important tool to use no matter which method of weight loss you choose. Simply put, keeping track of food intake and exercise increases weight loss success and it works for people on restricted diets as well as those who only want to keep track of calories. In fact, the more you journal, the more you lose.[69][70] There are many ways to keep track of the food you eat, but, spoiler alert, all require your input. The following are all easy and efficient ways to be accountable and control what you eat. Just choose the method that is easiest for you to use.

The Art Of Keeping Track

A food diary doesn't lie; it reveals how all your meals and snacks add up to help easily identify which eating habits are the most challenging to weight loss. Food journals also keep track of stress eating, weekend splurging, and desk and dashboard dining, not to mention cheating on portion sizes. I don't know about you, but sometimes I can't even remember what I had for dinner yesterday. For a food journal to work, consistency and accuracy are the two important factors that make it effective.

Consistency is important especially if you relax diet rules on the weekends or splurge on sweets while maintaining weight loss. It may also have the unexpected benefit of helping you skip the chips or the ice cream so you won't have to put it in writing.

Accuracy means keeping track of the exact weights and measures of food eaten. This is best accomplished when the recording is done at the time the food is eaten. Record food intake using paper or food logging apps but skip the photo apps. According to the 2SMART

Pilot Study, food photo apps are less reliable.[71] There is no denying that keeping daily food journals is time-consuming, but the time and effort needed to do it causes many people to slack off at a time when they should be doing anything but.

Keeping A Food Journal

Carefully choose from the methods available to you to find the one that works best with your schedule, technological aptitude, and lifestyle, because if it's not easy and convenient to keep up, you won't do it.

- **Pen and Paper** Using pen and paper always works, but technology can be more efficient with better options for more detailed supporting information. That said, a pen and paper journal is quicker and easier to master at the onset, but it does take time and that is the challenge. Looking up and recording calories, carbs, protein, and fats eaten is time consuming, but it can be done using info printed on the food label nutrition facts, websites like www.caloriecount.com, or reference books such as *Quick Check Food Facts* by yours truly.[72]

- **Web-Based** If pen and paper isn't your thing, web-based self-monitoring provides an on-line electronic diary, usually with built-in data bases with thousands of foods found in supermarkets and restaurants to make entries quick and easy. The recipe analysis features allow you to easily generate nutrition information from manually entered or downloaded recipes. These sites also provide ways to store lists of favorites and frequently eaten foods to make logging quicker. The feedback is instant and can be helpful in tailoring the next meal and snack to keep within daily goals. Some examples of web-based self-monitoring are www.myfitnesspal.com and www.loseit.com.

- **Mobile Devices** Smartphones and tablets all have access to software and apps to help you journal food intake. This gives you the convenience of having easy access to databases of calories, etc., when choosing what to eat in restaurants or on the run. Another useful tool included in some apps is the ability to analyze food for nutritional content by taking a photo of it. These nutrition-tracking apps using food photos is a growing field and their current reliability is questionable. Keep in mind that inputting the correct portion size is a must for the information to be accurate. As of this writing, these apps can't yet provide accurate analysis on mixed meals like stews. Some apps also provide recipes and shopping list capabilities that make preparing meals at home easier to pull off. Some even have the capability to reference the meals that worked well for you before to simplify menu planning.

Noom is an app that is lately leading the pack and boasts it has millions of users with a thousand more signing up every day for a free two-week trial. Noom is intended to be used for four months and among its unique features are:

- Its development team consisted of a dietitian, a nutrition researcher, and a psychologist

- The focus is on behavior change, which can lead to permanent weight loss

- No foods are off limits

- A questionnaire evaluates your goals, eating habits, and usual activity level to personalize specific calorie requirements

- Workout plans are available

- Offers support for emotional eaters and for navigating social events

- Daily messages keep you on track

- Access to coaches and a support group of members with the same common goals

In a study of over 35,000 Noom users, 77% lost weight.[73] Other smaller studies showed that users achieved a 5-7% loss of baseline weight. Noom is best matched to people who are self-motivated, can make food decisions on their own, don't mind paying the steep fee, and are comfortable using mobile device apps and the time it takes to learn them.

The bottom line is that recording daily food intake provides the best vehicle for self-evaluation, tracking progress, identifying challenges, and celebrating successes. In fact, any app that assists you in making better food decisions, whether at the market or heading for take-out, will improve your chances of keeping food intake in check. Using these self-monitoring tools will affect the lasting behavioral changes, which can result in permanent weight loss.

Shopping Apps

Again, pen and paper are old-school and reliable, but AnyList, Mealime, Out of Milk, and other shopping apps are available to help you navigate the grocery store aisles with ease. With Fooducate, simply scan an item's bar code to receive nutritional information and any fine print you would otherwise overlook (e.g., additives, preservatives, and *no-no* ingredients like high-fructose corn syrup). If you scan something that's not a wise choice, Fooducate will list healthier alternatives. For items without bar codes, like produce, just type in a search, and the app delivers the pros and cons, plus a quick-reference letter grade from A to D-. It also has the capacity to be on the lookout for and alert you to allergens, if necessary.

Dining Apps

Apps like Healthy Out and Healthy-Dining-Finder make it easy to eat out without undoing your diet. Healthy Out can locate restaurants in your area by cuisine or type of dish, including dietary preferences or restrictions (e.g., low-fat, low-calorie, gluten-free, heart-healthy, Atkins, Paleo, etc.). Both of these apps can note the healthiest choices on the menu, break down the nutritional information, and suggest modifications to make your order even healthier.

Mindfulness Apps

There are also apps to help with behavior change that address emotions, habits, and mindfulness. Am I Hungry? and Headspace-Mindful Eating provide help for weight loss, cravings, and binging by increasing awareness about food behaviors and feelings.

Wearable Fitness And Calorie Trackers

Pedometers, heart monitors, and other fitness trackers are all great tools for weight loss and wellness. Mobile apps that synch with wearable fitness trackers can also monitor sleep, physical activity, and heart rate for even more detailed health information. These categories of information are motivating as they provide the feedback on how well we are doing in advancing toward achieving a goal. This is essentially the pat on the back most of us need to stay motivated. This real-life tracking of physical activity and calories is a real eye-opener because most people, including health professionals, overestimate physical activity and underestimate calorie intake. These apps supply an opportunity to improve both intake and calorie burn, the winning formula in weight loss. We all know that when more calories are burned than consumed, weight is lost. But burning excess calories instead of storing them also means they don't contribute to further weight gain. New to the market is a device that is worn behind the ear, created by the University of Alabama, that counts chewing motions. It also has a camera that takes pictures of any food you are about to eat with feedback on the number of calories and the nutrients you literally have in front of you.

Wearable devices vary in reliability, complexity and price, so do your research because not all wearable devices are accurate. For example, when choosing an activity tracker, know that pedometers worn on the waistband or carried in a pocket are more accurate at counting steps than those worn on the wrist, as are some smart phone apps. Wrist wearables are popular, convenient, and adequate as activity trackers, but most are inaccurate at monitoring calories and tend to calculate and report more calories than really burned. In fact, a Stanford University study found most wrist fitness trackers were inaccurate about calories burned by 27 percent. One model in the study was off by 93 percent. Basing your calorie intake on misleading information can be detrimental. If the device ups your calorie goal to compensate for the calories it calculates you are burning, allowing you to eat more calories than actually being burned through exercise, ultimately it makes weight loss difficult or impossible. Some wearable devices feature an alert when you've been sitting or inactive for a long time, reminding you to get up and move, benefitting those with desk jobs and other sedentary lifestyles. Apps for your smartphone for the same purpose include Stand Up and BreakTime.

Clever Gadget

Another tool, HAPIfork helps slow your speed of eating by electronically measuring the time it takes to eat a meal. Because it takes the stomach 20 minutes to tell the brain when we have eaten enough, a fast eater consumes far more calories than needed to feel satisfied because of either taking bites too quickly or spending too little time chewing.

By the way, fast eaters also have more digestive issues and gastric reflux (heartburn) making the HAPIfork a useful tool when dealing with other eating-related health matters.[74] [75]

Fact: People who eat too fast are 42% more likely to be obese. Here are some suggestions for eating slower the low-tech way:

- Put the fork, spoon, or sandwich down between bites and chew and swallow every mouthful before picking up the utensil for the next bite

- Eat with your non-dominant hand, if you are a righty eat with your left, lefties eat with your right

- Use chopsticks for all foods

Nutrigenomics

It's the genes not the jeans. Yes, it's our genes that determine how we metabolize fat, proteins, and carbohydrates, and genetics may eventually be used to determine who will lose weight using which diet, but not yet. What we do know now is that there are both internal and external influences that can change how are genes are expressed. Nutrigenomics shows us how environmental factors (chemicals, temperature, and light, among others), food intake, and lifestyle all influence gene expression.

The genes we are born with may influence the tendency toward overweight/obesity but do not necessarily dictate a life destined to be overweight. By eliminating unhealthy food decisions and environmental exposures, the tendency to overweight can be suppressed instead of expressed.

If that sounds complicated, let me simplify. Nutrigenomics is the scientific study of how what we eat, how much we eat, and when we eat affects individual metabolism and weight. Think back to high school biology class when we learned how genes hold the information in code that make us who we are and influences how our body works. We are born with a unique genetic makeup, but it's our lifestyle and environment that determines which of these genes are expressed or activated. This is the reason your friend's diet doesn't work for you. It is also the reason why the one-size-fits-all diet recommendations bouncing all over the internet and media are a disappointment. Individuals respond differently because of genetic differences.

Genes are responsible for more than height and eye color; they also determine approximately 25% of a person's likelihood to become overweight/obese. Some experts even suggest that genes are responsible for up to 70% of the variables that determine which diet will work best for an individual given that genes are responsible for normal weight regulation, appetite, calorie intake, taste preferences, and how nutrients are processed. For example, a specific gene determines whether or not a person will gain weight from consuming saturated fats and another that reduces the risk of overeating. There are also genes that govern the tendency to choose sweet over fatty food or a preference for carbs instead of fats. Genes also influence the production of hormones like ghrelin, the appetite controller, and leptin, the fat storage manager. This means that body weight and body fat may be just as much a factor of genetic makeup as any diet and physical activity habits. In addition, genes determine an individual's response to exercise, including what type of exercise is most effective, how long it takes to recover, and which aerobic and strength-training strategies are most appropriate.

But the genes we are born with can be altered and, indeed, the genes affecting metabolism have been altered in obese individuals.

This is due, in part, by obesogens, compounds in the environment and in food that interfere with the natural body systems that keep weight constant. And, there is a gene that regulates sensitivity to obesogens. So, you see, it's not just about how genes influence energy balance, but also about how the environment influences those genes. Yes, a person can have genes for obesity and not be overweight due to environment and lifestyle. Alternately, a person can be overweight/obese without having the obesity genes.

To date, about 30 genes have been linked to BMI (Body Mass Index). One gene variant leads to obesity on a high-fat diet while another variant results in obesity with a high carbohydrate intake. One gene is known to increase the probability of weight gain with dairy consumption and another causes more weight loss with high fiber consumption. Another gene determines weight response to sweetened beverages, and yet another that is affected by fried foods. It has also been observed that the effects of some of these genes were either blunted or negated through physical activity. In chapter 6, I discussed how the gut microbiome affects weight. Well, genetics, in part, affects the microbiome, which then affects how each of us responds to a particular diet. This does not mean to run out and have your DNA tested. These discoveries are very recent and continue to develop. As I write this, researchers are seeking answers to why some people lose weight on high protein diets and others gain, what determines whether a person should choose a low-fat or low-carb diet regimen, and why people respond differently to identical diet and physical activity prescriptions.

The hope is that nutrigenomics will make it possible to design personalized gene-specific diets matching the exact foods and nutrients to individual health needs. We also look forward to personalized exercise regimens for maximum results. In the future, individuals struggling with weight may be given diet and lifestyle prescriptions using nutrigenomics that have the ability to influence gene expression.

Personalized nutrition has a long way to go before it is able to provide that type of dependable information. Don't jump on the media bandwagon just yet, but a DNA-specific grocery list could be the diet of the future.

Chapter 5:
Choosing Your Best Diet

As you can gather from this chapter title, it is not just a question of which diet is best, but which diet is best for you. Permanent weight loss success is not about restriction and deprivation. It is by healthy decision-making and practice. Keep in mind that there might not be only one way, but several that will get the job done.

It is common knowledge that there is no one way to lose weight, and that no one diet works for everyone. What is most effective for losing weight is to choose an eating plan that includes the foods you like to eat and allows for the lifestyle you enjoy. Your primary goal is to eat the appropriate number of calories for weight loss to occur. The choices you make on how to accomplish this calorie deficit must be made with your future life in mind because all food and behavior changes need to remain consistent and permanent for long-term success. If you can't make that commitment, you will lose and gain those same pounds over and over again.

Choose A Plan You Can Live With

Consider your needs. If following a list of food rules is not your thing, it stands to reason that you are unlikely to stick with a plan that relies on this method to reach your weight goal. On the other hand, if you are the type who says "Just tell me what to eat," you will benefit from a regimen with rules and restrictions. But people who do achieve permanent weight loss tend to rely on methods that take taste preferences, lifestyle, and health needs into account. If you haven't found success using strict diet plans, consider one that offers a more individualized approach.

Make sure your lifestyle, social life, travel, food availability, and exercise habits complement the diet protocol you are considering. Lifestyle factors and health issues play a larger role in weight loss than most people realize. That also goes for social activities that revolve around food and sharing meals with friends who have poor eating habits, which can lead to inferior food choices and overeating.

Also overlooked is having a job that keeps you chained to a desk for hours without a meal break or a chance to get up. Such a job is detrimental to your health and your weight. More and more often I hear from people who do not take time for lunch or they eat at their desk or skip meals altogether. Mindless eating and mild starvation are practices that always lead to overeating.

Switch Things Up

One way to increase success when using a restricted weight loss regimen is to switch between diets. This approach works because it reduces boredom and increases variety. Increased variety is especially important as it reduces the risk of nutrient deficiencies and also helps with suitable seasonal food choices or changes in your schedule. Rare is the method that helps you lose the first 20 pounds then continues to be effective enough to help you to reach your goal weight and then facilitate successfully maintaining the loss. Above all, choose a method that does not make you feel restricted or deprived. The best weight loss plan is one that teaches you how to effortlessly make the changes in your food choices seem natural, so they easily become habits. So, feel free to change methods, experimenting until you find one that seems like a natural fit. When you do, you will be able to take the weight off.

Do Not Rush The Process

Do not get frustrated if the pounds do not simply melt away. It may not be in the time frame you expected, but even losing a pound a month means being down 12 pounds in a year. A pound a week, a realistic goal, might not sound like much either, until you realize that is 52 pounds in a year. Just kicking a soda habit (one 12-ounce serving per day) and you will reduce calorie intake by 51,100 calories a year. Skipping one ounce of cheese a day will eliminate 36,400 calories in a year and roughly ten pounds. And, when you chose a method you can stick with, you will never see those pounds again.

Different Diets, Same Results

Comprehensive analyses of several weight-loss diets showed minimal differences in weight-loss results. Whether low-carb or low-fat, the average weight loss was 3.6 pounds in six months. Similar results were found in studies reported by the American Heart Association and the Obesity Society. This means that if diets are equally effective, then a fad diet is not the magic it's hyped up to be; it's simply the one trending at the moment. These fad diets are often not studied in a scientific and methodical way to determine how well they work, nor have they been around long enough to chart results.

A study published in February 2018, aptly named DIETFITS, clearly illustrates that after one year of dieting, participants had similar results whether they followed a healthy low-fat diet or a healthy low-carbohydrate diet, regardless of their gene patterns and insulin response to carbs. Important to note, however, is that both groups were instructed to reduce processed carbs and sugar and increase vegetable and fruit intake, but not to count calories. They were instructed to eat enough to not be hungry, which is an immensely helpful weight loss practice. The common factor here is the emphasis on healthy eating and vegetable and fruit consumption. This is because a diet high in vegetables and fruits is automatically lower in calories because those are foods with a naturally lower calorie density, a nod to the Volumetrics Diet (see page 54), which outperforms all other diets, but was never popular enough to be considered a fad. The DIETFITS study also accentuated that diet quality, not quantity, may be key to sustainable weight loss.[76]

Low Is Not The Way To Go

Neither low-carbohydrate nor low-fat in the extreme are healthy. Diets advocating low-carbohydrate eating encourage eating highly processed high-fat meats with bacon and beef jerky at the top of the list. However, following a lower carbohydrate diet when whole grains, fruits, and starchy vegetables replace foods high in unhealthy fats and overly processed grains is smart. Low-fat focused diets, on the other hand, push us toward food manufactured to be low in fat. The low-fat recommendations that were an attempt to curtail the growing overweight/obese population did not work because to re-make foods to be low in fat, processed carbs/sugar were added to make them palatable. Dieters snacked on low-fat brownies and large quantities of light ice cream and wondered why they were not losing weight. Healthy fats like nuts, seeds, and avocados are not only nutritious, but filling as well, highlighting the importance of fat in a weight-loss plan.

The take-home message here is to get off the SOFAS (<u>So</u>lid <u>F</u>ats and <u>A</u>dded <u>S</u>ugars), which include processed meats, cheese, desserts, and sugary drinks. And, don't forget to control portion size even with wholesome food and you'll lose weight and stay healthy.

PART THREE:
GETTING HEALTHY/ STAYING HEALTHY

Chapter 6:
Smart Eating = Smart Dieting

Eating smart means knowing not only which foods affect weight or how much food is a healthy portion, but gaining awareness of other factors that also influence weight gain as well. For example, researchers have now identified the negative impact that food additives, sugar substitutes, low quality fats, and food manufacturing practices have had on our weight. These substances have been identified as being toxic to the body and are being referred to as *obesagens*, compounds causing obesity. But, consuming more whole foods and limiting processed foods helps you avoid these toxins and compounds and their effect on your weight. In order to control your weight, you must be more selective about all your food purchases, and that includes take-out and restaurant meals. The best way to do this is to always read the ingredient list. A good rule of thumb is: if you see more than a short list or descriptive paragraph with words you struggle to pronounce, don't buy it. When selecting take-out, look for options made from fresh vegetables, lean proteins, and whole grains, with sauces, toppings, and natural flavors low in fat and sodium. It is also helpful to read the meal description on the menu before ordering to avoid the four Cs, creamy, crispy, crunchy and cheesy, to dodge the hidden fats. Maintaining a healthy gut can mean maintaining a smaller gut.

This chapter will set out ways you can adjust your eating habits and food choices to help you maintain a healthy weight along with high quality nutrition.

Believe The Science (not supermodels and celebrities)

Research results are definite on one thing: Weight loss is a complex subject. There are dozens of factors besides food that influence the success rate each one of us can achieve on any one diet, including genetics, sleep habits, physical activity, age, medications, and stress.

It's not only what we eat, but when, why, and how we eat, along with lifestyle choices that impact weight and the ability to lose or maintain it long term. Emerging science is investigating why certain diets affect individuals and populations differently. Although this research is still in its infancy, it proves that there is a need for personalized nutrition, especially for controlling obesity.

Organic Foods

This is one area that many people are struggling to understand, especially since more and more foods are labeled organic. It's difficult to know if they are better or worth the added price. Organic foods are those produced using methods that preserve the environment while avoiding chemicals and additives, such as pesticides, hormones, and antibiotics. This category of foods is also free of genetically modified ingredients (GMOs), which are increasingly present in our food supply.

GMOs And Pesticides

A GMO food is a food that has been altered by taking genes from one food source and incorporating it into the genetic makeup of an entirely different food source. Most GMO crops are developed to improve yield by increasing resistance to plant diseases and increasing tolerance to herbicides. Nearly 100% of the soybeans and corn grown in the U.S. are genetically modified.

Today's conventionally grown crops are often treated with chemical pesticides, including compounds such as organophosphates, carbamates, pyrethroids, and sulfonylureas. There is mounting evidence that pesticides disrupt the body's hormones and inhibit weight loss. Fruits and veggies high in pesticide residue can cause a rise in insulin, signaling the body to store fat. Pesticides, along with other toxins, have been identified as obesagens, substances that contribute to obesity. These toxins disrupt biochemical activities and block the normal functions of cells and organs, especially the gut. The body uses the gut wall as a first line of defense against harmful compounds and GMOs and most pesticides act as invaders, weakening the intestinal wall allowing these potentially damaging compounds (which do not naturally exist) to pass into the body.

To illustrate how pervasive these obesity-causing compounds are, consider corn. Ninety-three percent of the crop is GMO and conventionally grown using pesticides. Even if you make the decision to only eat organic corn, you still need to consider every form of corn you eat. Those obesagenic compounds are present in every single food containing corn, corn syrup, baking powder, tortillas, corn chips, cereal, popcorn, and even the ubiquitous food additive Xanthan gum. Don't forget that the animal proteins you also eat have been fed corn, genetically modified and full of chemicals, unless the meat label states grass fed or organic. The point here is not to avoid all these products, because you cannot, but you can choose to reduce the toxin load. Read food labels on all packaged processed foods and choose only those without corn and its derivatives. Avoid all foods with high fructose corn syrups (and beet sugars). Removing toxins and sugar is an easy way to eat smart by eliminating these known enemies in the weight war.

Unfortunately, organic foods can be both expensive and hard to find in some geographic areas. The Environmental Working Group (EWG) publishes a yearly list, called the "dirty dozen," of the produce with the highest contamination of pesticides.[77] A good, healthy eating strategy is to choose organic for foods you eat often, reducing the total amount of obesagenic compounds you consume.

Going organic is the best way to reduce exposure to pesticides, but, as I said, organic choices are not always available or affordable. The better strategy is to use the dirty dozen list as your guide to not eat those fruits and vegetables with the highest pesticide residues. Once you are familiar with this list, you can then make educated choices when buying organic for the foods you consume most often. The EWG also publishes on its website a list of the *clean fifteen* that identifies produce with the least pesticide residue that is conventionally grown and safe to eat.

Gut Health: The Microbiome

As if the compounds found in GMOs and pesticides altering our gut and hormones weren't scary enough, there's more to it than that. The ecosystem of both good and bad bacteria, along with the other organisms that coexist in the digestive system that are essential to preserving the immune system and health, is called the gut microbiome. The gut microbiome has a physiological influence on the body much like the hormones that regulate metabolism, blood sugar, and fat storage. The gut microbiome can also be quickly altered by diets high in fat and processed carbohydrates, medications, antibiotics, and even environmental factors. The disruption of healthy gut bacteria is also linked to obesity as well as gluten intolerance and depression. Because gut microbes have the ability to digest normally indigestible components of food, they provide additional absorbable calories, making it possible for an unhealthy microbiome to add otherwise avoidable calories, causing weight to be gained.

These little buggers not only influence weight and digestion, they also affect mental health by their ability to communicate with the brain. There is an amazingly strong connection between the gut and brain that is made possible through chemistry and the vagus nerve. Often referred to as an "information superhighway," neurotransmitters, the chemical messengers of the brain and nervous system, are mainly made by the gut microbes that have the ability to affect mood, including anxiety and depression. We know this because specific strains of bacteria are found more often in people suffering from depression. Additionally, depressed people also **lack** certain other strains of bacteria that correlate with depression. Another nod to the link between gut and mood is found in people with digestive disorders who suffer from higher rates of anxiety and depression. Scientists are finding evidence that a healthy microbiome can reduce stress and make a person feel calmer and happier.

The good news is that the microbiome can be preserved and restored with prebiotics and probiotics, foods and supplements that have the ability to support a healthy composition of organisms in the microbiome to restore gut health.

Probiotics are fermented foods that include yogurt, cheese, olives, sauerkraut, non-vinegar pickles, kefir, kombucha, miso and tempeh.

Prebiotics are foods that include bananas, raspberries, artichokes, asparagus, yams, chicory root, celery, beans, broccoli, leeks, and onions.

Eliminating or limiting animal protein, added sugar, salt, wheat, and processed foods while eating plant-based proteins, healthy fats, high fiber whole grains, fruits and vegetables is a good way to sustain gut health. Talk to a registered dietitian nutritionist for recommendations on appropriate prebiotic foods and probiotic supplements to restore a balanced microbiome.

Reliable Facts About Weight Control

While we wait for the science to provide all these answers, we still wonder what to eat to lose weight. Today we are sure that eating vegetables and fruits is one of the answers. Although we may not know everything at this point in time in the study of genomics, what we *do* know is that all research points to eating plant food as the solution to weight gain and disease management. No diet or pill required, just a regular trip to the produce section of the grocery or the local farmers market (wearing a fitness tracking device).

Use the following facts from science and professional weight loss experts to cut through the never-ending propositions and fads concerning weight.

✓ The eating of processed carbohydrates, sugar in snacks and drinks, fried and fatty foods and cheese, and not eating enough vegetables, fruits, and whole grains contributes to excessive weight

✓ The large portion sizes, served in restaurants, available in packaged foods, and what is plated at home encourages us to eat more than we need

✓ The abundance of food in our environment leads to eating even when we aren't hungry

✓ Low or no daily physical activity reduces calorie burn and leads to the storing of excess calories as fat

✓ Any diet that leads to deprivation and frustration cannot be sustained

✓ Sustainable weight loss is achieved by consistently practicing healthy habit-forming lifestyle and food behaviors

✓ Calories count, so reduce daily intake to lose weight

✓ Success with any one diet method is influenced by genetics, taste preferences, environment, readiness for change, medical issues, and exercise habits

✓ Eating protein is important while losing weight for preservation of muscle mass and metabolism, and it also helps maintain that fuller feeling longer

✓ Different carbs contribute in different ways to gaining belly fat

✓ A morning meal helps regulate weight by fueling the body to increase metabolism. It also controls cravings and appetite later in the day, and matches the circadian rhythm of energy needs and hormone levels

✓ Eating more foods with a high-water content means reducing calories without feeling hungry or deprived

✓ Eating all meals within a 6-to-12-hour window is an effective weight and fat loss strategy

✓ Limit exposure to chemicals, preservatives, and food additives that alter how the body uses calories and stores them as fat

✓ Drink more water instead of high-sugar juice and soda to eliminate calories from beverage choices

✓ Don't eat when you aren't hungry, to avoid calories from unnecessary snacking and emotional eating

✓ Don't skip meals, which slows metabolism and causes weight gain

✓ An unhealthy gut microbiome can cause overweight/obesity

✓ Genes influence metabolism and weight regulation by determining the processing of nutrients and non-nutrient compounds in food, and by determining the effectiveness of exercise, and whether fats or carbs are friends or enemies

✓ Keep a food and exercise journal to avoid underestimating food intake or overestimating physical activity

✓ Stop mindless and distracted eating to fully experience the taste and texture of food; eating in front of the television or while doing tasks leads to overeating

Adopt the Habits of Weight-Loss Superstars

If scientific research isn't your thing, get motivated by reading about the weight-loss success of those who have lost significant weight and kept it off for a long time. The National Weight Control Registry tracks over 10,000 of these amazing individuals.[78] These high achievers have no specific method or diet in common, but all used diets that relied on calorie restriction. What they did have in common, though, was in how they are keeping weight off:[79]

✓ Everyone eats a lower fat diet, 25-30% of total calories, despite the latest research finding that dietary fat is not the enemy in the battle of the bulge.

✓ They all count calories and adhere to a daily calorie goal by eating portion-controlled low-calorie dense foods

✓ Every person self-monitors, keeping a food journal, for example

✓ All engage in high levels of physical activity, especially planned exercise, about 60 minutes every day to boost metabolism

✓ Their behavior is consistent, practicing healthy habits, along with sticking to mealtimes and exercise schedules

✓ All eat breakfast

✓ All make sure they sleep well

✓ All practice mindful eating, an awareness of how various foods affect feelings, thoughts, and physical sensations by tuning in to temperature, texture, and taste while eating.

There you have it—the secret to long-term weight loss success.

Chapter 7:
The Challenges of Successful Dieting

Before you start on any diet plan, however, it is important to remember that replacing old habits takes work. Whether it is in time and energy, or emotional, mental, or physical effort, dieting is challenging. On a positive note, taking on a challenge is good because it leads to change. When looking for long-term weight loss or wellness, food behaviors are what need to change. These changes are always easier when you are ready to undertake the self-reflection (i.e., keeping a food journal) necessary to help you analyze your habits to identify the ones that need to change.

Overeating

It is important to address the reasons why you overeat. For many of us it is because we were raised to clean our plates, or to celebrate successes with big meals and sweets. For others it was to soothe hurt feelings by eating, by being treated to an ice cream sundae instead of a hug. Emotional eating with its roots in stress, boredom, and loneliness can also be a reason for unhealthy food decisions. The treat we got as a child may now be the box of cookies we indulge ourselves with to unwind after a hard day at work, or perhaps it's a porterhouse steak with all the fixings when eating out. The habit of soothing or celebrating with food often leads to the habit of overeating.

If this is you, once you identify why this happens, you will be able to devise an effective plan, perhaps choosing a different activity that doesn't include food to celebrate, or to soothe, reward, or combat boredom. Inseparable from the emotions that drive us to overeat are the feelings of guilt, low self-esteem, and shame that follow. When overeating or another bad food decision leads you to more overeating, it's time to change the behavior. Unfortunately, countless dieters respond to making poor food decisions by vowing to start dieting again on Monday, which never works. Real change can only come about when the poor choice is addressed immediately. The better solution is to take a walk, plan a healthy meal to follow, or plan a weeks' worth of healthy options. Then, without shame and with self-worth intact, devise a well-thought-out plan for the next time the same situation arises, eliminating the tendency to overeat.

The Role of Willpower

Many of us have been misled to believe that being unsuccessful is a direct result of lacking willpower. Willpower, the ability to delay gratification for a future reward, is not infinite. In fact, willpower is a muscle that tires with use. When you consider all that you need to resist on a daily basis from dealing with your boss or spouse to spending above your budget, it is no small feat to have enough willpower in reserve to limit calories. Add to that the severe calorie restriction of many diets that in effect limit the fuel that the willpower muscle needs to function. Severe calorie restriction also triggers low blood sugar levels, which impact decision making. In other words, consider that maybe it's the dieting itself, with the resulting undereating and poor food choices, that is the reason or at least a contributing factor to overeating. Since it is common for dieters to skip meals while dieting to save calories to justify an evening overconsuming or to under-eat all week to overindulge all weekend, all that accomplishes is to set up a cycle of undereating/overeating. This then causes metabolic and emotional changes that in turn challenge hunger, satiety, and the management of food intake.

Only by removing the diet mentality of placing blame on the lack of willpower, and truly engaging in the act of self-evaluation as to the real causes of your poor food behaviors, can this issue be addressed.

Eating What You Enjoy

Another challenge to dieting is whether or not the rules you are expected to follow match your food preferences and food availability. When you analyze the make-up of your daily food intake, be sure to note if you are always reaching for carbohydrates or choosing high-fat foods or regularly including cheese and bread in meals and snacks. Note if you eat a significant amount of protein at every meal. When you have these facts, you can compare your findings to the diet prescription you are considering and have a much better chance of success. Be truthful with yourself because a person who fills each meal and snack with carbs will have a difficult time on Atkins and Ketogenics. The one who struggles with vegetables will have a hard time sticking with Volumetrics, Weight Watchers, and Whole30.

The diet you choose must match your food preferences or the struggle to avoid the foods you enjoy will be too great a challenge to your weight-loss efforts.

Mindless Eating

Where you eat is as much a factor of weight as what you eat. Eating out and ordering take-out, eating at your desk or in front of the TV all affect your food intake. Large portions coupled with the distractions of tasks, video games, and television lead us to overconsume an estimated additional 150 calories at each meal due to mindless eating.

We also tend to eat more in the presence of food. Meetings around a conference table full of food, or snacks on the kitchen counter encourage eating simply because of the availability. We aren't eating from hunger, it doesn't even have to be a food we really enjoy—it's simply within reach and difficult to resist.

Dining companions also influence what and how much we eat. Overeaters, overweight or thin, encourage overeating in others around them. Dieters are less likely to stick to the rules of the diet plan when eating with or near overweight individuals unless they are careful to keep their goals in mind.

Motivation—Know Yours

Another key factor that challenges weight loss and weight maintenance is knowing what is motivating you to lose weight. Never underestimate the impact of the why. Your motivation is a key component because it encompasses the amount of effort and conviction you must have when the going gets tough (and it will). It is hard to make food and lifestyle changes, but identifying why you want to lose weight increases the chance of success. Maybe you are not able to make friends or travel. Maybe you want to dress in more stylish clothes or have the energy to keep up with the grandchildren. These are a few of the most common motivators, but maybe yours is different. What is important is that you know your why. Know what really matters to you and if it matches your current lifestyle. Know what you want that you don't have.

Timing is Everything

Lastly, think about timing. Perhaps your past dieting efforts weren't successful because it wasn't the right time. Life gets in the way. We can get derailed by family, jobs, and other responsibilities that fill the calendar or overwhelm our thoughts and emotions. Therefore, be honest when you ask yourself if you are now up for the challenge.

Chapter 8:
Successful Weight Maintenance

Maintenance is key. Reducing daily calorie intake and/or increasing physical activity may be in order since your body is burning fewer calories at a lower weight with the same activity level.

Modify Calorie Intake

Significant weight loss reduces the need for energy, which translates to needing fewer daily calories. In fact, researchers found that after a 20-pound loss from a calorie restricted diet, the body needs an average of 100 calories less per day, a small number of extra calories that slowly add up to a ten-pound gain over the course of a year. So, it is easy to see how diligently sticking to a weight loss plan is no guarantee of successful weight maintenance.

Here again is when a food journal is helpful because it will highlight when portions have increased, or splurges are more frequent. Daily food logs with accurate weights and measures provide an honest assessment of backslides into old food behaviors. It may be time to re-evaluate your daily calorie goal, however, and adhere to the general rule that total calories should not fall below 1,200 per day.

Time for New Rules

This may be a good time to choose a new diet plan. Alternative ideas in food choices and meal composition may be just what you need to achieve a weight-loss break-through and prevent boredom and frustration, making it easier to keep your resolve to stick to your new habits. Also, a change in diet plan can alleviate nutrient deficiencies, improving the quality and nutrient density of food selections. After all, weight maintenance is easier for a healthy, well-nourished body. The Mediterranean and DASH diets are proven excellent weight maintenance plans.

Commit to Exercise

The best strategy for maintaining your new weight is exercise. Remember, you must burn as many calories as you eat to maintain weight and burn more calories than you eat to lose weight.

Knowing how much physical activity it takes to burn the calories in specific foods is helpful for making good food choices. Known as exercise equivalents, these are based on weight and exercise duration and intensity.

The American Council on Exercise provides an exercise equivalent calculator on their website.[80] Just to give you an example of how this works, let's use Taco Bell Beef Taco Salad as an example. To burn those 760 calories, a 170-pound person would have to climb stairs for 1 hour 15 minutes. A 250-pound person would need to walk for 3 hours and 20 minutes at a casual pace to use up those same calories instead of storing them.

Exercise equivalents should help you to first consider how much effort it takes to burn those calories before you eat them to influence your decision to eat that food or the portion size you select. Exercise equivalents also help in planning how much exercise is needed for splurges and holiday eating. If and when you see the number on the scale rising or feel your clothes tightening, do not despair. It is much easier to address a small weight gain than a large one. Increase physical activity to burn more calories, making it easier to lose any weight gained from the temporary increase in calorie intake.[81]

Physical activity revs up and optimizes metabolism and a faster metabolism means the ability to burn off calories, keeping the weight off. Common to all long-term losers is their commitment to an exercise regimen. It is recommended that 60 minutes a day be devoted to exercise, either all in one session or spread throughout the day—it doesn't matter as long as it is at least one hour in total. Increasing or preserving metabolic rate is an important factor in the long-term sustainability of the weight lost (look up what happened to The Biggest Loser Competitors).[82]

A frequently asked question is about the best type of exercise to rev up metabolism. One strategy is to increase muscle building exercises because muscle is more metabolically active; it burns more calories. Another strategy for breaking through a plateau is to change your exercise routine. Muscles have memory, so if you keep the exercise workouts the same, over time, they are less challenging to the body leading to fewer calories burned. For example, if you have been walking on the treadmill for the past 6 months, switch to the bike, elliptical or aerobic dance class. If you prefer only walking, try high intensity interval sessions or walk on the beach or up hills in the neighborhood. Another strategy to turn up the burn is with activities of daily living, time spent on self-care and chores, creating short bursts of High Intensity Incidental Physical Activity (HIIPA); consider it an exercise snack. Examples would be climbing stairs, walking to a meeting, house cleaning, gardening, parking far away from your destination, and carrying groceries at a pace that would elevate your breathing and heart rate. You can fit in a short burst of activity on your way to the bathroom at work or putting away the laundry at home. International researchers agree that HIIPA promotes weight loss and weight management without devoting time to a planned exercise regimen. HIIPA is ideal for people who are physically capable of activity but are short on time or without the opportunity to exercise.

Plateaus Are Not as Bad as You Think

Weight maintenance is as essential to weight management as weight loss because once the target weight is achieved, it doesn't magically stay there. In fact, most studies document that weight loss slows at the six-month mark and regain of lost weight is common at twelve months on fad diets.

Sadly, no matter how weight is lost, most people regain it. Typically, weight loss plateaus, or stops, after 6 months on any weight loss plan. A plateau is when, despite diet and exercise adherence, no weight is lost for 2-3 weeks. Far from indicating failure, or the inability to lose any more weight, it's simply Mother Nature at work. The brain and body strive to maintain weight much like they maintain a steady body temperature. Both are self-preservation systems referred to as homeostasis. The science is that the brain overrides the body even when it has loads of fat to shed. The brain keeps the body within a specific weight range called the set-point, even when the body is overweight—and the brain will fight to stay at that set-point even when weight loss is the healthiest option.

This made sense during human evolution when food was scarce, and the system preserved weight to keep the individual alive. Today this same set-point causes weight loss to plateau and seems more counterproductive than helpful. But if you consider the weight loss plateau as a healthy holding pattern, giving the body a chance to regroup and establish a new lower set-point for the brain and body to comfortably maintain, you are on the right track.

Maintaining your new weight during a plateau is cause for celebration because maintaining hard-won successful weight loss is more than a steppingstone, it's a victory. Here's why. Energy needs decline with lower body weight. The leaner body has a lower metabolism and that means it burns fewer calories performing all activities. This energy gap means eating less or burning more just to maintain the lower weight.

Metabolism regulates energy use and is influenced by behavioral and environmental factors. Behavioral factors include food choices and portion size, the amount and type of physical activity, and sleep quantity and quality. Environmental factors include availability of appropriate food, social surroundings, and opportunity for physical activity.

Stay in Control When Life Gets in the Way

Despite our best behaviors and best intentions, life often gets in the way. We can't avoid stress, social situations, celebrations, travel, and family obligations that often present obstacles to healthy food behaviors, but we have control of our responses to them. It takes mindfulness, effort, and planning to sustain healthy eating habits.

First, think it through. When weight loss or weight maintenance become challenging, you don't need to abandon nutrition and exercise goals. Identify the challenge or potential problem. Be as detailed as you can about the situation that leads to unhealthy choices. Think through potential solutions and choose one. Devise a plan that will result in a healthy outcome. For instance, you find yourself spending more time on the road and resorting to fast food stops when you get hungry. Your clothes are starting to feel a bit snug. You can avoid the rest stops but you know you won't be able to avoid the hunger. You decide to prepare and pack appropriate meals and snacks at home before the trip.

Apply mindful eating techniques to increase awareness of negative behaviors and non-food activities. If your social calendar is full of events that include food, try paying more attention to the people you are with and your surroundings, and putting less emphasis on the food in front of you. The party atmosphere and the conversations then entertain you instead of the food. If you are emotionally eating, find an activity that does not include food to soothe or reward.

Splurge and enjoy. Yes, you read that right. When you make a conscious decision to eat a big meal or take a second helping of dessert, don't let guilt and negative self-talk detract from your enjoyment of it. Savor the experience, being present and fully mindful of the pleasing sensations including the taste and texture of the food. The food experience will be more satisfying when feelings of deprivation and remorse are removed. When you detract from enjoying the food, your desire for that food will stay strong and unfulfilled, and you will need more to feel satisfied. Chocolate may be a good example since many people deny themselves. If you allow yourself an ounce of chocolate a day, without negative thoughts or feelings, you are less likely to overdo it when faced with a whole bar or box of chocolates.

There Is No Finish Line

Some diet methods take time to produce results while others feel like a race to reach a finish line, a magic number on the scale. But, unfortunately, for most people, there isn't a moment in time when attending to your food decisions and lifestyle choices ends. Not if you want to preserve the weight you have fought hard to reach.

Weight maintenance also requires a plan of action and vigilant adherence to it. The plan can include specific rules like the diets previously discussed or a conglomerate of principles chosen from several strategies that helped you reach your goal weight.

Weight maintenance does not mean that the number on the scale will always register your ideal weight. The truth is there is no perfect number indicating a person is at a perfect weight. Besides, perfection is a goal, not a reality. When the scale gets stuck on a number or registers weight gain, it is too easy to begin negative self-talk. However, negative talk leads to negative effort, and without the diligence with which you have been following your weight loss plan, the result can be regaining the weight you worked so hard to lose. Before you panic or reach for the bag of candy, pause to think and plan. Get back on track as soon as possible. Just as you had a plan to lose the weight, now is the time to plan on keeping it off.

Holidays, vacations, and other occasions that alter schedules and food availability, or add physical or emotional stress, can lead to weight gain. It is disheartening see the results of eating large meals and extra desserts, but do not despair. Address the weight gain as soon as it is evident by following the strategies that were most successful in the past. Keep in mind, it is easier to lose recent weight gain than to wait until the body has adjusted to it. And addressing a five-pound gain is easier than waiting until you are carrying around an additional 10-15 pounds. On the other hand, you may even find you don't experience holiday and vacation weight gain when healthy eating and lifestyle behaviors are habits.

The Truth is...

For those of you who are looking to lose weight and want some magic potion or plan that will melt the fat off by Friday, that pipedream is unattainable. The simple fact is that there is no magic combination of foods or one food group that will make you lose weight. Where weight loss is concerned, I'm afraid there is no quick fix. The truth is that you did not miraculously wake up one morning being overweight. It happened over time, and therefore will be shed in the same way, over time. Quick weight loss tends to be unsustainable and rapid weight loss is not good for your health. Anyone can choose a drastic weight loss method and lose 5 pounds in a week. If your goal is to fit into your clothes for a party come Saturday, go for it. But more than likely, those 5 pounds will return quickly and probably with a few more. And you then begin the search for the next quick fix to try.

You can be successful at losing weight and, yes, weight loss can be permanent. But, like many other good things in life, it will take time, effort, and practice. Think about how many times you fell when learning to ride a bike before you learned how to balance and steer. You probably had more than one person teaching you as you advanced from tricycle to training wheels to a 10-speed, but once you learned to ride, you never forgot. Dieting is like riding a bike. Once you find the eating plan that works for you and suits your lifestyle, it is yours for life. It's the one you can comfortably live with. Instead of focusing on the foods to avoid, you focus on the delicious and healthful food choices you can eat. Eventually the healthier foods will naturally crowd out the unhealthy ones and you will never feel deprived or restricted.

Start by replacing just one unhealthy food and you'll see results. Once this happens you feel more confident, and able to make another change, then another, until healthy eating becomes a habit. I will always remember the client who expressed joy over discovering how many healthful foods he was able to eat and actually preferred once he tried them. He was happy to eliminate the unhealthy foods from his diet, which he was really only eating out of habit. He was able to both enjoy eating and maintain a healthy weight.

Whatever dieting method you choose and however many pounds you lose, be sure to celebrate your success, whether it is one pound or five. Search and try a few methods until you find the one that feels most compatible with your food preferences and lifestyle. That way, eating won't be challenging, and the results will be most satisfying.

Yes, you can win your weight loss battle when you find the method that works best for you.

References

1 https://www.niddk.nih.gov/health-information/health-statistics/
   overweight-obesity

2 http://www.slideshare.net/alicehenneman/portion-distortion

3 https://www.cdc.gov/nccdphp/dnpa/nutrition/pdf/portion_size_
   research.pdf

4 https://www.cdc.gov/nccdphp/dnpa/nutrition/pdf/portion_size_
   pitfalls.pdf

5 Johnston, B. C., Kanters, S., Bandayrel, K., Wu, P., Naji, F., Si-
   emieniuk, R. A., ... & Jansen, J. P. (2014). Comparison of weight
   loss among named diet programs in overweight and obese adults:
   a meta-analysis. *Jama*, *312*(9), 923-933

6 Ebbeling, C. B., Feldman, H. A., Klein, G. L., Wong, J. M.,
   Bielak, L., Steltz, S. K., ... & Ludwig, D. S. (2018). Effects of a
   low carbohydrate diet on energy expenditure during weight loss
   maintenance: randomized trial. *bmj*, *363*, k4583

[7] Robert C. Atkins, MD., Dr. Atkins Diet Revolution (New York: David McKay Company, Inc., 1972)

[8] Larosa, J. C., Fry, A. G., Muesing, R., & Rosing, D. R. (1980). Effects of high-protein, low-carbohydrate dieting on plasma lipoproteins and body weight. *Journal of the American Dietetic Association, 77*(3), 264-270

[9] Dansinger ML, Gleason JA, Griffith JL, Selker HP, Schaefer EJ. Comparison of the Atkins, Ornish, Weight Watchers, and Zone Diets for Weight Loss and Heart Disease Risk Reduction: A Randomized Trial. *JAMA*. 2005;293(1):43–53

[10] William Davis, MD, Wheat Belly (New York: Rodale Books, 2011)

[11] Glenn A Gaesser, Perspective: Refined Grains and Health: Genuine Risk, or Guilt by Association?, *Advances in Nutrition*, Volume 10, Issue 3, May 2019, Pages 361–371

[12] David Perlmutter, MD., Grain Brain (New York: Little, Brown Spark, 2013

[13] https://www.webmd.com/diet/video/truth-about-gluten

[14] http://celiac.org/celiac-disease/diagnosing-celiac-disease/screening/

[15] Ye, F., Li, X. J., Jiang, W. L., Sun, H. B., & Liu, J. (2015). Efficacy of and patient compliance with a Ketogenic diet in adults with intractable epilepsy: a meta-analysis. *Journal of Clinical Neurology, 11*(1), 26-31

16 Bueno, N., De Melo, I., De Oliveira, S., & Da Rocha Ataide, T. (2013). Very-low-carbohydrate ketogenic diet v. low-fat diet for long-term weight loss: A meta-analysis of randomized controlled trials. *British Journal of Nutrition, 110*(7), 1178-1187

17 Ello-Martin, J. A., Ledikwe, J. H., & Rolls, B. J. (2005). The influence of food portion size and energy density on energy intake: implications for weight management–. *The American journal of clinical nutrition, 82*(1), 236S-241S

18 Stelmach-Mardas M, Rodacki T, Dobrowolska-Iwanek J, Brzozowska A, Walkowiak J, Wojtanowska-Krosniak A, Zagrodzki P, Bechthold A, Mardas M, Boeing H. Link between Food Energy Density and Body Weight Changes in Obese Adults. *Nutrients.* 2016; 8(4):229

19 Raynor, H. A., Looney, S. M., Steeves, E. A., Spence, M., & Gorin, A. A. (2012). The effects of an energy density prescription on diet quality and weight loss: a pilot randomized controlled trial. *Journal of the Academy of Nutrition and Dietetics, 112*(9), 1397-1402

20 Rolls, B. J. (2017). Dietary energy density: Applying behavioural science to weight management. *Nutrition bulletin, 42*(3), 246-253

21 Buckland, N. J., Camidge, D., Croden, F., Lavin, J. H., Stubbs, R. J., Hetherington, M. M., ... & Finlayson, G. (2018). A low energy-dense diet in the context of a weight-management program affects appetite control in overweight and obese women. *The Journal of Nutrition, 148*(5), 798-806

22 Rolls, B. J., Drewnowski, A., & Ledikwe, J. H. (2005). Changing the energy density of the diet as a strategy for weight management. *Journal of the American Dietetic Association, 105*(5), 98-103

23 http://www.artfido.com/blog/photographic-series-showing-what-200-calories-looks-like-in-different-foods

24 http://robbwolf.com/what-is-the-paleo-diet/meal-plans-shopping-guides/

25 http://www.youtube.com/watch?v=BMOjVYgYaG8

26 http://www.eatright.org/resource/health/weight-loss/fad-diets/should-we-eat-like-our-caveman-ancestors

27 https://blogs.scientificamerican.com/guest-blog/the-true-human-diet/

28 Megan A. McCrory, Bruce R. Hamaker, Jennifer C. Lovejoy, Petra E. Eichelsdoerfer, Pulse Consumption, Satiety, and Weight Management, *Advances in Nutrition*, Volume 1 Issue 1, November 2010, Pages 17–30

29 Mellberg, C., Sandberg, S., Ryberg, M., Eriksson, M., Brage, S., Larsson, C., ... & Lindahl, B. (2014). Long-term effects of a Paleolithic-type diet in obese postmenopausal women: a 2-year randomized trial. *European journal of clinical nutrition*, 68(3), 350

30 Klempel, M. C., Kroeger, C. M., Bhutani, S., Trepanowski, J. F., & Varady, K. A. (2012). Intermittent fasting combined with calorie restriction is effective for weight loss and cardio-protection in obese women. *Nutrition journal*, 11(1), 98

31 Harvie, M. N., Pegington, M., Mattson, M. P., Frystyk, J., Dillon, B., Evans, G., ... & Son, T. G. (2011). The effects of intermittent or continuous energy restriction on weight loss and metabolic

disease risk markers: a randomized trial in young overweight women. *International journal of obesity, 35*(5), 714

32 Harvie, M., Pegington, M., Mattson, M. *et al.* The effects of intermittent or continuous energy restriction on weight loss and metabolic disease risk markers: a randomized trial in young overweight women. *Int J Obes* 35, 714–727(2011)

33 Varady, K. A. (2011). Intermittent versus daily calorie restriction: which diet regimen is more effective for weight loss? *Obesity reviews, 12*(7), e593-e601

34 Jordan, S., Tung, N., Casanova-Acebes, M., Chang, C., Cantoni, C., Zhang, D., ... & Gainullina, A. (2019). Dietary intake regulates the circulating inflammatory monocyte pool. *Cell, 178*(5), 1102-1114

56 Rangan, P., Choi, I., Wei, M., Navarrete, G., Guen, E., Brandhorst, S., ... & Abdulridha, M. (2019). Fasting-mimicking diet modulates microbiota and promotes intestinal regeneration to reduce inflammatory bowel disease pathology. *Cell reports, 26*(10), 2704-2719

36 University of Southern California. (2019, March 6). Fasting-mimicking diet holds promise for treating people with inflammatory bowel disease: Clinical trial shows reduction of inflammation in humans; diet appears to reverse Crohn's and colitis pathology in mice. *ScienceDaily.* Retrieved August 24, 2019

37 Henst, R. H., Pienaar, P. R., Roden, L. C., & Rae, D. E. (2019). The effects of sleep extension on cardiometabolic risk factors: A systematic review. *Journal of sleep research*, e12865

38 Al Khatib, H. K., Harding, S. V., Darzi, J., & Pot, G. K. (2017). The effects of partial sleep deprivation on energy balance: a systematic review and meta-analysis. *European journal of clinical nutrition, 71*(5), 614

39 Anton, S. D., Moehl, K., Donahoo, W. T., Marosi, K., Lee, S. A., Mainous III, A. G., ... & Mattson, M. P. (2018). Flipping the metabolic switch: understanding and applying the health benefits of fasting. *Obesity, 26*(2), 254-268

40 Zaman, A., Rynders, C., Steinke, S., Tussey, E., Kealey, E., & Thomas, E. (2019). SAT-096 Later Timing of Energy Intake Associates with Higher Fat Mass in Adults with Overweight and Obesity. *Journal of the Endocrine Society, 3*(Supplement_1), SAT-096

41 Chaix, A., Zarrinpar, A., Miu, P., & Panda, S. (2014). Time-restricted feeding is a preventative and therapeutic intervention against diverse nutritional challenges. *Cell metabolism, 20*(6), 991-1005

42 Jakubowicz, D., Barnea, M., Wainstein, J., & Froy, O. (2013). High caloric intake at breakfast vs. dinner differentially influences weight loss of overweight and obese women. *Obesity, 21*(12), 2504-2512

43 Juliane Richter, Nina Herzog, Simon Janka, Thalke Baumann, Alina Kistenmacher, Kerstin M Oltmanns, Twice as High Diet-Induced Thermogenesis After Breakfast vs Dinner On High-Calorie as Well as Low-Calorie Meals, *The Journal of Clinical Endocrinology & Metabolism*, Volume 105, Issue 3, March 2020, dgz311

44 Hoertel, H. A., Will, M. J., & Leidy, H. J. (2014). A randomized crossover, pilot study examining the effects of a normal protein vs. high protein breakfast on food cravings and reward signals in overweight/obese "breakfast skipping", late-adolescent girls. *Nutrition journal*, *13*(1), 80

45 https://www.ewg.org/news/videos/ewg-and-pesticides-dirty-dozen

46 www.whole30.com

47 Shai, I., Schwarzfuchs, D., Henkin, Y., Shahar, D. R., Witkow, S., Greenberg, I., ... & Tangi-Rozental, O. (2008). Weight loss with a low-carbohydrate, Mediterranean, or low-fat diet. *New England Journal of Medicine*, *359*(3), 229-241

48 Mente, A., de Koning, L., Shannon, H. S., & Anand, S. S. (2009). A systematic review of the evidence supporting a causal link between dietary factors and coronary heart disease. *Archives of internal medicine*, *169*(7), 659-669

49 Martínez-González, M. Á., De la Fuente-Arrillaga, C., Nunez-Cordoba, J. M., Basterra-Gortari, F. J., Beunza, J. J., Vazquez, Z., ... & Bes-Rastrollo, M. (2008). Adherence to Mediterranean diet and risk of developing diabetes: prospective cohort study. *Bmj*, *336*(7657), 1348-1351

50 Valls-Pedret C, Sala-Vila A, Serra-Mir M, et al. Mediterranean Diet and Age-Related Cognitive Decline: A Randomized Clinical Trial. *JAMA Intern Med*. 2015;175(7):1094–1103. doi:10.1001/jamainternmed.2015.1668

51 Lassale, C., Batty, G. D., Baghdadli, A., Jacka, F., Sánchez-Villegas, A., Kivimäki, M., & Akbaraly, T. (2019). Healthy dietary indices and risk of depressive outcomes: a systematic review and meta-analysis of observational studies. *Molecular psychiatry*, *24*(7), 965-986

52 Crous-Bou, M., Fung, T. T., Prescott, J., Julin, B., Du, M., Sun, Q., ... & De Vivo, I. (2014). Mediterranean diet and telomere length in Nurses' Health Study: population based cohort study. *Bmj*, *349*, g6674

53 http://www.nhlbi.nih.gov/health/public/heart/hbp/dash/new_dash.pdf

54 https://www.nhlbi.nih.gov/health/health-topics/topics/dash/getstarted

55 Huang, R. Y., Huang, C. C., Hu, F. B., & Chavarro, J. E. (2016). Vegetarian diets and weight reduction: a meta-analysis of randomized controlled trials. *Journal of general internal medicine*, *31*(1), 109-116

56 Dawn Jackson Blatner, RD, LDN, The Flexitarian Diet (New York: McGraw-Hill, 2009)

57 https://dawnjacksonblatner.com/books/the-flexitarian-diet/flexitarian-diet-recipes/

58 Lowe, M., Miller-Kovach, K., & Phelan, S. (2001). Weight-loss maintenance in overweight individuals one to five years following successful completion of a commercial weight loss program. *International Journal of Obesity*, *25*, 325-331

[59] Dansinger, M. L., Gleason, J. A., Griffith, J. L., Selker, H. P., & Schaefer, E. J. (2005). Comparison of the Atkins, Ornish, Weight Watchers, and Zone diets for weight loss and heart disease risk reduction: a randomized trial. *Jama, 293*(1), 43-53

[60] Tsai, A. G., & Wadden, T. A. (2005). Systematic review: an evaluation of major commercial weight loss programs in the United States. *Annals of internal medicine, 142*(1), 56-66

[61] Davis, L. M., Coleman, C., Kiel, J., Rampolla, J., Hutchisen, T., Ford, L., ... & Hanlon-Mitola, A. (2010). Efficacy of a meal replacement diet plan compared to a food-based diet plan after a period of weight loss and weight maintenance: a randomized controlled trial. *Nutrition journal, 9*(1), 11

[62] Wadden, T. A., Foster, G. D., Letizia, K. A., & Stunkard, A. J. (1992). A multicenter evaluation of a proprietary weight reduction program for the treatment of marked obesity. *Archives of Internal Medicine, 152*(5)

[63] Seimon, R. V., Wild-Taylor, A. L., Keating, S. E., McClintock, S., Harper, C., Gibson, A. A., ... & Liu, P. Y. (2019). Effect of Weight Loss via Severe vs Moderate Energy Restriction on Lean Mass and Body Composition Among Postmenopausal Women With Obesity: The TEMPO Diet Randomized Clinical Trial. *JAMA network open, 2*(10), e1913733-e1913733

[64] Rolls, B. J., Roe, L. S., Beach, A. M., & Kris-Etherton, P. M. (2005). Provision of foods differing in energy density affects long-term weight loss. *Obesity Research, 13*(6), 1052-1060

[65] www.splendidspoon.com

66 https://ginacucina.com/

67 Evelyn Tribole, MS, RDN, CEDRD-S and Elyse Resch MS, RDN, CEDRD-S, FIAEDP, FADA, FAND, Intuitive Eating (New York: St. Martin's Publishing Group, 1995, 2003, 2012, 2020

68 Arterburn, L. M., Coleman, C. D., Kiel, J., Kelley, K., Mantilla, L., Frye, N., ... & Cook, C. M. (2019). Randomized controlled trial assessing two commercial weight loss programs in adults with overweight or obesity. *Obesity science & practice*, 5(1), 3-14

69 Harvey, J., Krukowski, R., Priest, J., & West, D. (2019). Log often, lose more: electronic dietary self-monitoring for weight loss. *Obesity*, 27(3), 380-384

70 Patel, M. L., Hopkins, C. M., Brooks, T. L., & Bennett, G. G. (2019). Comparing self-monitoring strategies for weight loss in a smartphone app: randomized controlled trial. *JMIR mHealth and uHealth*, 7(2), e12209

71 Dunn, C. G., Turner-McGrievy, G. M., Wilcox, S., & Hutto, B. (2019). Dietary self-monitoring through calorie tracking but not through a digital photography app is associated with significant weight loss: The 2SMART pilot study—A 6-month randomized trial. *Journal of the Academy of Nutrition and Dietetics*

72 Amy Newman Shapiro, RDN, CDN, CPT, Quick Check Food Facts (New York: Barron's Educational Series, Inc, 2016)

73 Chin Sang Ouk & Keum, Changwon & Woo, Junghoon & Park, Jehwan & Choi, Hyung & Woo, Jeong-Taek & Rhee, Sang. (2016). Successful weight reduction and maintenance by using a smart-

phone application in those with overweight and obesity. *Scientific Reports*. 6. 34563. 10.1038/srep34563

[74] Hermsen, S., Mars, M., Higgs, S., Frost, J. H., & Hermans, R. C. (2019). Effects of eating with an augmented fork with vibrotactile feedback on eating rate and body weight: a randomized controlled trial. *International Journal of Behavioral Nutrition and Physical Activity, 16*(1), 90

[75] https://www.hapilabs.com/product/hapifork

[76] Gardner, C. D., Trepanowski, J. F., Del Gobbo, L. C., Hauser, M. E., Rigdon, J., Ioannidis, J. P., ... & King, A. C. (2018). Effect of low-fat vs low-carbohydrate diet on 12-month weight loss in overweight adults and the association with genotype pattern or insulin secretion: the DIETFITS randomized clinical trial. *Jama, 319*(7), 667-679

[77] https://www.ewg.org/

[78] http://www.nwcr.ws/

[79] Paixão, C., Dias, C. M., Jorge, R., Carraça, E. V., Yannakoulia, M., de Zwaan, M., ... & Santos, I. (2020). Successful weight loss maintenance: A systematic review of weight control registries. *Obesity Reviews*

[80] https://www.acefitness.org/education-and-resources/lifestyle/tools-calculators/physical-activity-calorie-counter

[81] Klaas R Westerterp, Physical activity and body-weight regulation, *The American Journal of Clinical Nutrition*, Volume 110, Issue 4, October 2019, Pages 791–792

[82] https://www.nytimes.com/2016/05/02/health/biggest-loser-weight-loss.html

CPSIA information can be obtained
at www.ICGtesting.com
Printed in the USA
JSHW040213170121
11003JS00001B/5